CANDIDA
Killing So Sweetly

Proven Home Remedies to
Conquer Fungus and Yeast Infection

Earth Clinic Presents...

CANDIDA:

Killing So Sweetly

By Bill Thompson

An Earth Clinic Publication

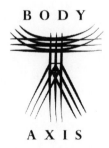

BODY

AXIS

Body Axis, LLC.
Atlanta

DISCLAIMER
The preparation and publication of this book has been undertaken with great care.
However, the book is offered for informational purposes only and cannot be taken
as a substitute for professional medical prevention, diagnosis, or treatment. Please
consult with your physician, pharmacist, or health care provider before taking any
home remedies or supplements or following any treatment suggested by anyone
within this book. Only your health care provider, personal physician, or pharmacist
can provide you with advice on what is safe and effective for your unique needs or
diagnose your particular medical history.

Visit us online at:
www.bodyaxis.com
www.earthclinic.com

Printed in the United States of America

FIRST PRINTING: 2013
ISBN-978-0-9828963-8-9

Candida – The Invisible Disease

This essential book argues and presents both an evidence-based research view and a testimonial view of Candida in order to assimilate hard facts about how this organism behaves as a pathogen, how infections arise. It also presents several successful remedies and methods, with aftercare, that ensure riddance and infection prevention with no continual return of the yeast/fungal infection.

Dedication

My special tribute and thanks to those healers such as Ted from Bangkok (aka Parhatsathid Napatalung), Walter Last and Dr Jennifer Daniels as well as my respect to those honest doctors and researchers, such as Dr Orion Truss, Dr William G Crook, Dr William Shaw, Dr Burt Berkson, Dr Guy Abraham and Dr David Brownstein as well as so many others, who have all proven that compassionate medical curiosity is certainly alive and well. These people truly understand and appreciate the (forgotten) meaning of the word "cure". Without their honest open knowledge and contributions, this book would have been quite impossible to write.

Acknowledgements

My grateful thanks to Deirdre Layne, Daniel P. Kray and everyone at Earth Clinic for all their wonderful help and patience in advising, promoting and supporting me in this endeavour.

Table of Contents

AUTHOR'S PREFACE

One of the prime reasons for writing this book has been that, as an ex-systemic candida sufferer whose deliberate study of candida has been ongoing for several years now, I have learned that modern medicine still seems to have such an inadequate research viewpoint or understanding of candida as a yeast/fungal disease—both from the diagnostic and treatment points of view on how to actually deal with and cure candida problems.[12,16,17] Candida, in whatever form, I regard as a particularly insidious and non-trivial disease that can be quite as difficult to identify as to cure because it is such a robust and adaptable pathogen form.

My own background is simply as a layman who has had the great misfortune to have been infected by candida and who has cured this disease himself using a particular multi-remedy methodology that was highly successful. I have also helped advise other people with candida problems and seen the remedies in this book work successfully to help others resolve their own candida problems. Let me admit right now that I am not a qualified doctor nor have I any research or PhD qualifications. But I happen to regard myself as a very logical man who is simply looking for honest answers and who spends most of his spare time these days reading medical and alternative research papers and testimonials just to find out exactly what really is effective to cure candida and other auto-immune diseases. Well some folks like collecting stamps or they like gardening as a hobby—but my hobby, if you like, is reading and deciphering medical research. I do this because, for me, reading these research papers is better than reading any adventure story or thriller novel. I love the main plot (incurable candida) and I love the real heroes (honest, independent researchers and healers).

Another main reason for writing this book is to simply and in plain words define and explain what candida is as a pathogen as well as to present several candida remedies – based upon my own experience and all the *true evidence* – that will actually work successfully to help cure all the different forms of candida: localized candida (arising in the skin, uterus, sinus etc.), intestinal candida and the more virulent and difficult fungal form which I had—systemic or disseminated candida.

This book will verbally and visually show the reader or candida sufferer exactly what candida is as a pathogen—how robust and adaptable it is as a dangerous parasite and how it behaves and spreads throughout the body; how candida has two distinct and differing biological dimorphic forms; how a candida infection is normally associated with a plethora of other pathogens and diseases, which gives rise to all the many differing and confusing symptoms for candida. That's why no two candida sufferers will ever have exactly the same symptoms – and consequently why candida is such a very difficult disease to both properly identify and cure – which is perhaps the best reason I can think of as to why doctors and the medical profession are so inept at properly and accurately diagnosing both early and later stage candida problems.

The two best and most revealing books I have ever read on candida as a disease are *The Missing Diagnosis* by Dr Orian Truss and *The Yeast Connection* by Dr William G. Crook. Both authors were honest medical doctors who laid out radically different methods of cure for candida using diet as their main approach. That's to say that they completely departed from the medical profession's usual antifungal/antibiotic drugs approach in their advice and treatment protocols for candida. These two books, although written in the 1980s, are still very relevant as highly useful background reading for candida sufferers and are still well worth referencing today.

To be absolutely clear, this book will not advise any form of patented drugs or antibiotics to cure your candida. The approach used in the anti-candida protocols in this book is holistic as well as dietary, incorporating the broad use of body-friendly nutrients and herbs as well as an essential diet along with detoxing in a multi-protocol system that aims to successfully kill off all forms of candida (together with all other associated pathogens) and raise the immune system back up to healthy levels. An optional liver and kidney protection protocol with a vitamin and mineral regimen will help the user recover health more quickly. A simple but essential anti-candida diet is also involved with the protocol and is fully described.

I am also writing this book in great appreciation of the remedies that I mainly used to cure my own candida problems. The remedies from *The Main Anti-Candida Protocol* given in this book are certainly not my own—most of the remedies herein, together with all due praise, belong to Ted from Bangkok (aka Mr Parhatsathid Napatalung) who regularly advises and posts on the Earth Clinic website.

If, over the years, you have been to the doctor innumerable times to find a cure for your candida problems – of whatever form – and if you still have this ongoing disease years later or, indeed, if you believe that you have some indefinable and debilitating *mystery illness* where the doctors cannot pinpoint any causative disease or pathogen with their blood, urine or stool tests—then this book will help you. I cured my own systemic candida problem seven years ago, including curing a raft of other symptoms and associated diseases like psoriasis, eczema, constipation, low thyroid, jock itch, chronic athlete's foot, brain fog, heart arrhythmia, low energy, digestion problems, insomnia etc. by just following *The Main Anti-Candida Protocols* laid out in this book. To date (seven years later) my candida, including all of the other horrible symptoms mentioned, has never returned. That said, this book will also give you a much clearer grounding and wider understanding about candida and how to get rid of this awkward disease swiftly and for good—including advising preventative aftercare and diet, by just using the advice and protocols given within this small book.

However, if you are just looking for a quick, easy and convenient cure for your awful candida problems, then this is probably the wrong book for you. From what I already know about candida as a disease, there simply is no quick and easy cure for serious candida problems where you just take two pills in the morning and two pills in the evening and that's it, you're suddenly cured. Curing candida means breaking bad eating habits and strictly following a healthier diet and lifestyle. When you ask yourself the question, "Why do I have candida?" then the answer must be, as one of the prime causes, what you have been putting in your mouth every day for the last few decades. So you will stand little chance of curing your candida unless you follow a strict and careful diet. A multitude of specific nutrients and remedies are also advised in the *Main Anti-Candida Protocol* for use on a daily basis and all the good reasons for their use will be fully explained. The protocols in this book aim for a cure and not just to treat or accommodate your fungal disease. Therefore using this protocol and achieving success will also require a degree of personal mental focus, dedication, determination and willpower by the candida sufferer wishing for a cure. In other words, the outcome is really up to you. There are no short-cuts. This book will also attempt to explain and lay out all the convincing reasons why candida is so difficult to diagnose, let alone to cure.

Furthermore and for greater clarity, this book will, for the most part, avoid using fancy scientific language meant to show you how incredibly clever I am. The whole point of this book is to put this important information out there clearly as a definite, proven and useful aid to help ordinary people like you and me understand, identify and successfully resolve their own difficult fungal disease—*Candida: Killing So Sweetly* (2013).

Bill Thompson
San Fernando
The Philippines
March 2013

DEFINITION OF TERMS

candidemia: A candida infection that has spread into the blood, tissues and organs of the body (older usage).

candidiasis: Used as a general term for a candida infection.

disseminated candida: Synonymous with candidemia and systemic candida.

dimorphic: Applied to an organism that has two distinct living forms.

fibrin: A form of glycoprotein that is a main constituent in candida yeast/fungal biofilms.

fibrinolytic: Applied to an agent that removes or inhibits the formation of fibrin.

invasive candidiasis: Synonymous with candidemia and disseminated candida.

mycelial form: Fungal form.

saprophyte: An organism that feeds only off dead organic matter.

saprophytic: Applied to an organism that only feeds off dead organic matter.

parasite: An organism that feeds only off host cells and/or host nutrients.

pleomorphic/polymorphic: Used to denote several distinct forms of the same organism. Dimorphism is an example of pleomorphism.

CHAPTER 1:

Understanding the Invisible Enemy

"Know thyself, know thy enemy;
a thousand battles, a thousand victories."
—Sun Tzu (Art of War)

In beginning to understand candida fully as a disease it is enlightening to examine the behaviour of candida as a pathogen and it is, perhaps, initially most useful to consider the morphology or the biological structure and make-up of this pathogen.

Candida can exist in two distinct forms—it can exist as a yeast and also as a fungus. It is also quite important, as a starting point, to realize that many other dangerous pathogens co-exist in the lower human intestines along with candida in what's called a symbiotic state. Symbiotic means that the invading organism benefits as well as the host from the dual relationship. The invading pathogen does no real harm to the host because the host's immune system and healthy body state are fully capable of maintaining a healthy defensive environment for the host, thus suppressing invading organisms, thereby preventing these pathogens from morphing or changing into a more dangerous or damaging pathogenic form. There are also many other potentially dangerous pathogens that continually and naturally inhabit our lower intestines – such as E. coli, Giardia, Salmonella, H. pylori etc. – that co-exist in a suppressed and controlled state as harmless symbionts within the lower intestinal area, which can only ever be attributed to the actual strong health state of the human host.

"My doctor says that he (she) doesn't believe in chronic candidiasis" is a statement that many patients have relayed to me. The latest textbooks continue to treat yeast as more of a nuisance than as a significant cause of chronic ill health, the principal exception being the instances of deep (formerly "systemic")

1

candidiasis associated primarily with diseases of the cells of the immune system itself (HIV, leukemia, lymphoma, etc.)."
—Dr Orion Truss

It is also well known through research that candida can exist in a human host in its fairly harmless and innate localized state as a yeast. Indeed, the candida yeast form can be found in the lower intestines in the majority of our human population. But being the less virulent yeast form, coupled with the strong immune system and good health state of the human host, this is unquestionably what acts to continually suppress the candida yeast form (as well as other dangerous pathogens already inhabiting the lower gut) and prevents it from morphing into the much more virulent, dangerous and invasive fungal form.[37] As a direct parallel and as further evidence if you like, cancer cells are created in the body every single day and it can only be the strong health state of our bodies and immune system that prevents the cancer from gaining a foothold then dominating and ultimately metastasizing (spreading) rapidly throughout our tissues and organs.

Another perhaps simpler example might equally demonstrate my point. I'm sure most readers have experienced or noticed what I am about to describe. I've noticed that whenever there is a flu epidemic in my own area, there are people who never get the flu—even during the height of an epidemic. Similarly, there are also people who catch every single round of cold or flu that comes their way and then some. What could be the reason for this? It is only when the human body's immune system is in such a hugely weakened, suppressed or defenseless state that diseases like cancer, candida and even flu and colds can easily proliferate and spread throughout our bodies either slowly or like wild-fire (as quickly our health state deteriorates) with such ease. It therefore seems to me quite reasonable to further suggest that the susceptibility and speed of spread of these diseases – including candida – is directly proportional to and highly dependent upon anything that will erode, suppress or destroy the human body's immune system, which further acts to demean the human body's critical, optimum health state.

Progressive Weakening of the Immune System

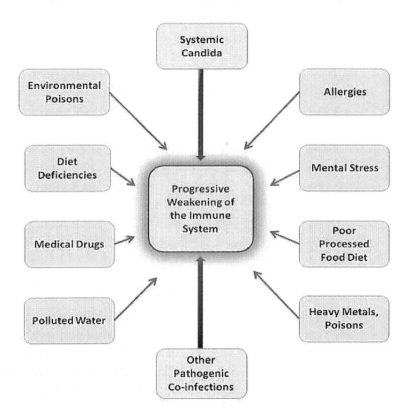

Let me further dispel some other myths about candida. Candida is not a bacteria and not a virus – it is a yeast/fungus – so you should not approach the treatment or eradication of candida as anything resembling or related to the normal treatment for viral or bacterial problems. You are making a big mistake if you do not heed this warning. If bacteria and viruses are the regular enemy troops that attack our bodies and our immune system, then you should regard candida as their Special Forces or as a highly competent guerrilla terrorist force that can hide in your body using biofilms; candida can breed with the host cells, thereby easily adjusting to medicines; candida can cause cravings in its host for its favourite food: sugar. It is both a saprophytic yeast and a fungal parasite with a dual form[37-40] that is always associated with many other pathogenic forms and diseases[15,19,32,35] and one that uses superior chemical warfare to continually weaken our immune system via its waste products, which act to poison and wreak havoc in our bodies with excessive levels of aldehydes, alcohols and poisonous proteins including tartaric acid and arabinose (a five-carbon aldehyde sugar).[8,9,10] Knowing what I now know about candida and the effects of their waste products, I would far rather be infected with bacteria or a virus than from any fungus like candida.

> *"In the 1940's Candida was found in only three per cent of autopsies, now the figure is nearer thirty per cent. There are, of course, other factors that can cause dysbiosis - the contraceptive pill, steroids and other drugs, radiation treatment and chemotherapy - but the main culprits are, without doubt, antibiotics."*
> *—Walter Last (Candida and the Antibiotic Syndrome)*

Now to the next fungal myth. I've read many web blogs and testimonial descriptions from people who make hugely wrong assumptions when treating their own candida problems. The result of this incorrect thinking or strategy is that they are completely unable to make any headway at all in curing their own candida problem. I will give you some examples along the way to help illustrate this important point more clearly, because if your thinking is initially all wrong on the how-tos of curing candida, when you start to try to heal yourself – and candida being the clever, camouflaged and confusing guerrilla pathogen that it so naturally is – then I personally doubt if you will ever stand much chance of succeeding.

As a general example of the above problem, let's say that Janet has had a uterine candida problem for over five years. She has tried just topical meds recommended by the doctor and has also tried innumerable alternative topical candida therapies to get rid of her own vaginal candida but she is completely unable to get rid of it. It therefore never goes away or, if the candida does go away, it always seems to return eventually with a vengeance; i.e. the candida was just hiding and was never cured in the first place. Other factors, like a continuous bad diet and lifestyle, will also play their own part in encouraging the spread and persistence of candida. The above example applies equally to people who have localized candida such as skin problems, oral candida, vaginal candida, fungal nasal problems etc. and is a typical example of the incorrect thinking that I have read on many health blogs.

The problem is that the above thinking and cure strategies are all wrong in the first place. If you have already tried all sorts of topical remedies to cure your own localized vaginitis, thrush or candida skin problems and have always failed, then what must be the real problem? If all the topical remedies failed to work – time and time again – then what is the logical reason for this failure? The reason must be that your apparently localized candida problem cannot be just a topical, localized problem but is instead caused by a more serious and deeper candida infection that has arisen inside your body—from the systemic candida or fungal form that has infected your blood, organs and tissues. In other words, that your local sinus problem or uterine yeast problem or skin problem or the fungal nasal problem that you have is *actually just a symptom of the systemic or disseminated candida form itself.* Therefore you will not be able to cure your local problem by using just topical remedies and you will have no option but to take the proper steps to rid your internal systemic candida infection first if you ever want to make any headway at all with your localized candida problem.

As proof of this, my own systemic candida symptoms were brain fog, low thyroid, eczema, psoriasis, jock itch, constipation, chronic athlete's foot (I had this problem for over 20 years), digestion problems, insomnia, lethargy, low energy, racing heart and vertigo. When I set about curing my own candida I never even bothered to topically treat any of my localized fungal skin problems with anything. But after I had completely cured my own candida using the protocols, every single one of my other problems or "systemic candida symptoms" just disappeared—including all my local fungal skin problems. The main caveat here is, never immediately assume that your uterine yeast problem or your candida skin problem or oral candida problem or your intestinal candida etc. is just a localized problem. The likelihood of your localized problem being caused by the systemic candida form also greatly increases if you have had your localized candida problem for years and years. And if the topical or local therapies completely fail to get rid of it, you must therefore conclude that your localized candida problem has actually arisen because of a deeper internal, systemic candida infection and treat it accordingly in order to finally achieve successful candida riddance from your own body.

> *"The most common manifestations [of candida], in addition to anxiety and inappropriate depression, may include: bloating, diarrhea, constipation, indigestion, vaginitis (aggravated by antibiotics and birth control pills), urethritis, cystitis and other skin problems (acne, hives, diaper rash, oral thrush, athlete's foot, jock itch, nail infections), chronic fatigue, chemical intolerance to food and inhaled chemicals, headaches (migraine and sinus), nasal, sinus, and bronchial allergies, menstrual disorders, decreased libido and impotence, premenstrual tension, and impairment of short term memory and concentration as well."*
> –Dr Orian Truss

Now to another unfortunate candida fallacy that is very prevalent. Having read so many blogs and research articles concerning candida problems, it has become disturbingly clear to me that many ordinary people still believe that if they can get rid of their candida from just their intestines then they will be cured. More bad thinking. I've already made clear the point that candida has two distinct forms[37-40]—the more docile yeast form and the highly virulent fungal form. It is certainly true enough to say that usually the intestines are the initial seat or internal throne of candida (as the yeast form) for a short while. The yeast form exists characteristically as a *saprophyte*—it feeds and obtains nutrients from dead organic matter, in the intestines or the uterus for example. The more dangerous and robust fungal candida form is a proper parasite that feeds directly off host tissues and host nutrients. After changing into the more virulent fungal systemic form, candida therefore morphs into a completely different beast. It suddenly becomes highly mobile as fungal spores and is then able to spread easily and at will throughout your body into your blood, organs and tissues where it dominates and similarly spreads further into the body. So, deciding on a misbegotten strategy of just getting rid of the candida from your intestines as the cure, when you may have the virulent systemic fungal form already so widely disseminated throughout your own body (outside your intestines) must be regarded as a particularly unrewarding strategy. What usually happens is that you may indeed get rid of the candida from your intestines for a short while, but it always comes back in full force because you haven't even attempted to get rid of the systemic form (which requires a different and more specific multi-protocol approach) already so widely prevalent throughout your body. After you get rid of the candida from just the intestines, what usually happens is that the systemic form that still resides in the blood, organs and tissues of your body then eventually re-infects and re-populates these areas and the candida simply spreads back into the intestines after a period of time – it comes back – and you will have made little progress in ultimately curing your own candida problem.

It has become very apparent to me that both lay-people and even some doctors still believe this myth about getting rid of candida only from the intestines as an all-around cure for your candida. Nothing could be further from the truth if you already have the systemic or disseminated fungal candida form. As a result of this mistaken approach and for too long many ordinary people, as well as some doctors, remain in the mindset that candida is a trivial intestinal disease that can be easily cured by taking a few pills in the morning and a few pills in the evening. People with candida who also believe that candida is a simple and trivial disease are, in my opinion, wishing for a cure upon a very far and distant star indeed.

Right now I can imagine certain readers mumbling the obvious question, "Well then, how can we test and confirm whether we have the systemic candida form in our bodies or not?" A good question and the truth of it is that modern medicine has no accurate method to test for ordinary intestinal candida (the yeast form), let alone a suitable test to identify systemic candida (fungal form). Doctors will only ever use stool, blood and urine tests to check for candida—and these tests are notoriously inaccurate. There is a new antigen test for candida that is extremely expensive, which is why most doctors don't recommend it. So the truth of it is that there is no standard, accurate test for systemic candida in our bodies. I have also read several recent reviews and studies on candida diagnosis and treatment that even admit that early diagnosis via the current medical testing methods for candida are indeed sadly inadequate.[12-17]

So what can we do?

The first thing you should do, if the doctors are unable to help you or you are dissatisfied with their approach or diagnosis, is take responsibility for your own candida problem and start investigating and researching this disease for yourself. Learn all about the enemy within your body and make up your own mind. And since the main anti-candida protocols defined in this book are designed to cure all the different forms of candida – including the localized, intestinal and the systemic forms – I would simply advise that you do the anti-candida protocols described herein as the answer and remedy.

As a further aid and useful test for candida, Orian Truss and William Crook were medical doctors and competent authors who wrote ground-breaking books about candida. They also recognized that the modern medical profession was fairly inept at both diagnosing and treating candida. After all, this was the main reason why Orian Truss titled his book *The Missing Diagnosis*. So, in order to help people identify their own candida problems, both authors brought out notable questionnaires that worked off a points system to determine whether an individual had candida or not and these questionnaires are online for free and easily accessible today.

> *"Candida is responsible for flooding the system with an accumulation of toxic acetaldehydes. Acetaldehydes are known to poison tissues – accumulating in the brain, spinal cord, joints, muscles and tissues."*
> *–Dr Stephen Cooter, 'Beating Chronic Illness'*

Another remarkable misconception that some people have about candida is the oddly-held belief that their candida infection is no more dangerous or difficult to get rid of than the common cold. After all that I've just described in the short section above, it should have become quite clear to the reader that candida is indeed a clever and robust pathogen – with complex associations and behavioural relationships with other pathogen species – that is highly adapted for survival and is confusing and difficult to recognize and cure as a consequence. In its initial stages, candida infection may barely be noticed. But if the candida infection is left unattended to spread freely for years or even decades, it then becomes a highly dangerous organism capable of completely destroying your quality of life or worse. A sudden stress event – either mental or physical – such as a death in the family of a loved one or perhaps a food poisoning event or excessive antibiotics over a period of time can certainly be enough to suddenly accelerate the grip that candida already has on your body, with odd new symptoms or even new diseases or allergies erupting and arising because of the swift drop in the capabilities of your immune system. In other words, candida is one of the most patient, adaptable and opportunistic of all the pathogens that are known. So this organism should really be feared and respected because of its considerable abilities to adapt and learn from its own host environment.

Root Causes of Candida

Candida, as well as bacterial pathogens like H. pylori, Salmonella, E. coli etc., can always be found in the lower intestines of most humans. But normally, in a healthy body, the intestinal immune system is easily able to suppress the spread of candida.

Candida can also infect the body topically as in skin candida, uterine candida, nasal candida, oral candida etc. It is also important to realize, because of candida's dimorphic behaviour, that any initial topical candida infection can easily give rise, over time, to a deeper fungal infection in the blood, tissues and organs where candida eventually spreads throughout the whole body. Conversely, it is also quite important to realize that an internal systemic candida infection can give rise to a multitude of topical or localized problems as symptoms of the systemic form.

The root causes of candida are defined below:

•Frequent use of antibiotics and other medical drugs such as steroids, chemotherapy, the contraceptive pill etc.[58]

•Heavy metals, chemical processing and other agri-poisons in the modern processed food diet, which always lower the capabilities of the immune system.

•Lack of essential nutrients – minerals, vitamins and amino acids – in the diet.

•An already weakened or compromised immune system.

Candida Symptoms

For me, this section has been one of the most difficult areas to write because candida has so many associations, by way of co-infections, with other diseases and pathogens; which quite naturally will affect the overall expression of symptoms for candida. I have read much research on these associations and they are profuse! So, in all honesty, there are no hard and fast symptoms that can easily identify candida as the disease you have—because there are so many crossover symptoms with other diseases. And because so many diseases are and can be associated with candida, candida symptoms will therefore get all jumbled up with the symptoms of other associated diseases like IBS, GERD, Fibromyalgia, Myalgic Encephalomyelitis (ME), Chronic Fatigue Syndrome, Colitis, Parasites, Low Thyroid, Crohn's Disease, Lupus, Rheumatoid Arthritis, Psoriasis—on and on ad infinitum. In order to quickly demonstrate the extent of symptoms, here is a reasonable but abbreviated list of possible symptoms for candida:

•Stomach problems
•Intestinal digestion problems
•Lethargy, low energy, brain fog, low thyroid
•Depression

- Multiple skin problems (e.g. persistent athlete's foot, psoriasis, eczema, rash)
- Rheumatoid arthritis, myalgia or tissue pain
- Constant constipation or diarrhea
- Allergies or food sensitivities
- ENMT problems that persist (e.g. white tongue, itchy ears, sinusitis, rhinitis, dry cough)
- Persistent uterine yeast or vaginitis problems
- Persistent UTI problems
- Prostate problems
- Weight gain or rapid weight loss
- Suffered recent and serious mental or emotional trauma such as a death in the family
- Suffered a physical trauma such as food poisoning or other debilitating disease
- Parasite problems

Other related problems and symptoms can also be associated with candida such as slowed reflexes, depression, lethargy and apathy, decreased mental energy, anxiety, fatigue, obsessive-compulsive disorder, PMS and breast swelling/tenderness in women, headaches, memory loss, hives, seborrhoea, skin rashes, bloating, nasal congestion, infertility, ocular "floaters," pelvic pain, loss of libido, neuritis, arthritis, Crohn's disease, hypoglycaemia, schizophrenia, anorexia nervosa, lupus, hyperactivity, behaviour problems, learning problems and autism.[7]

The above list is much reduced and generalized to save some room. You can find other lists of candida symptoms on the internet and in other candida books that run into a couple of pages!

My own personal opinion about the above huge symptom list is that it will be of little help to any candida sufferer and will, perhaps, only ever tend to further confuse. Instead, if you're not sure whether you have candida, I would take the Candida Self Test (see the next section) and complete William Crook's online candida questionnaire[64] which, at no cost, will at least give you a result and confirm, fairly accurately, whether you do indeed have a candida problem or not.

Self-Testing for Candida

Candida is a very confusing disease whose symptoms can be so easily confused with a plethora of other health problems. Furthermore, modern medicine has quite a poor reputation for properly diagnosing and confirming early stage candida. So the best way to confirm whether you have candida is to take the following rudimentary tests for yourself.

The Candida Spit Test

The spit test should be performed first thing in the morning before you brush your teeth and before you rinse your mouth. Spit into a full glass of water. The saliva will initially sit on top of the water but after about 15 minutes you may see thin strands of spit extending down like small tentacles towards the bottom of the glass. If this is the case then you are probably positive for candida.

Other positive indications might be cloudy saliva that will sink to the bottom of the glass within a few minutes or particles that slowly sink or suspend below the saliva glob. These are colonies of yeast that band together to form strings.

If, after this period of time, your saliva shows none of the above attributes then you most likely are negative for candida.

The White Tongue Test

This test just involves inspecting your own tongue. If the surface of your tongue is unusually white or blotchy white instead of a healthy pink colour, then it is likely that you have, at the very least, oral candida. This may also indicate, as a symptom, the presence of intestinal or systemic candida.

William Crook's Online Questionnaire

This questionnaire may be found online (See the *Resource Index*[64] for the link). The useful questionnaire works off a points system and is fairly accurate at diagnosing candida.

Antibiotics and Candida

It is a well known fact that, in the treatment of candida, the use of antibiotics will always work to actually help spread the candida and even make it more virulent.[56,57,58] Most of the alternative healing community already knows and fully accepts that antibiotics, used for whatever period of time, are useless and even dangerous to use against candida; and certain medical doctors (though by no means all) also know and accept this as fact. This problem is referred to as The Antibiotic Syndrome.[58] Whenever antibiotics are used over any period of time it is already proven through research that antibiotics destroy all the beneficial bacteria in the gut thus actively causing dysbiosis – an intestinal imbalance of good and bad bacteria – allowing candida as well as other dangerous pathogens complete free rein to spread up into the upper intestines, eventually to dominate and extend their havoc throughout our bodies. Furthermore, candida is not affected or reduced at all by antibiotics.

Alexander Fleming discovered penicillin in 1928, for which discovery he received the Nobel Prize in 1945. He made the discovery when he noticed that a mold had contaminated and developed in one of his Petri dishes containing bacteria and that there was an area around the penicillin mold that was completely free of bacteria. Hence the birth of penicillin and the whole antibiotics industry. But few people will make the connection here. Penicillin – and all other antibiotics – are in most cases derived from molds. Molds are very closely related to yeast and fungus. So how can any antibiotic, which has been developed from a fungal organism to act against bacteria, kill another fungal organism existing in the same genus or family? In other words, neither penicillin nor any other current antibiotic will ever act to kill or eradicate any fungus, mold or yeast disease. I hope this is now very clear. Do not ever take any antibiotics if you have candida—doing so will only ever act to encourage the spread of candida and further reinforce the downward health spiral in your own body.

"The increase in incidence of acute yeast vaginitis has been estimated to approach 1500%, with the percentage of cases of acute vaginitis caused by yeast increasing from 25% in 1940 to 90% in 1965."
—Dr Orian Truss

It is also most interesting to note that there have been no new antibiotics invented or manufactured since 1987. Why is this a fact? The hard reasons for this are because modern research and modern medicine now fully realize that they are losing the war against bacteria by using antibiotics. They have simply given up inventing any new antibiotics because bacteria are so easily able to adjust to any antibiotic – both old generation or new generation – so quickly.

It takes about ten years to properly research and invent a new antibiotic drug and it can cost the drugs company up to $200 million up front to prove the efficacy and safety of a single antibiotic (or indeed for any other drug) for acceptance by the FDA.

Unfortunately, it has also been estimated that any new antibiotic that comes onto the medical market today has now a useful medical life expectancy of only one year before bacteria are able to adjust to it and it becomes ineffective—which is not enough time for any drugs company to reclaim their vast moneys spent on research or to enable them to make a useful profit.

As a result of the above facts, modern medicine's current arsenal of anti-bacterial drugs is rapidly becoming useless and depleted. It is well known that bacteria can breed in resistance to any antibiotic within a fairly short time period. MRSA or Golden Staph and C. diff are classic examples of this. Bacteria can also hide in biofilms, thus completely avoiding any beneficial antibiotic effect while also avoiding attack by the host immune system.

Much more disturbing are concerns raised in some recent medical research articles from The Lancet. Apparently, bacteria are now able to produce a certain specific enzyme called *The New Delhi-metallo-*

beta-lactamase-1 enzyme. This enzyme – also referred to as NDM-1 – has the unique ability to cleave antibiotic molecules, rendering their effect useless against bacteria. What is much more disturbing is that the bacteria that are already able to manufacture this NDM-1 enzyme are, somehow, passing on this ability to other and different bacterial species.[53] So, for example, whereas in the old days if you had an E. coli infection then antibiotics could easily be used to kill the bacteria causing the problem. But now, if E. coli has learnt this ability to produce the NDM-1 enzyme, then E. coli cannot then be stopped or cured effectively with any antibiotic, and so the future prospects of dangerous E. coli pandemics will necessarily rise (especially in hospitals) with a huge increase in mortality rates, since antibiotics are now so useless against any bacteria capable of manufacturing the NDM-1 enzyme. Currently, the NDM-1 enzyme has already been found in Enterobacter, Pneumonia and UTI bacteria and it seems to be steadily spreading to other bacterial species. So far this enzyme has jumped and spread across 14 separate species of bacteria. And if this NDM-1 enzyme is predicted to spread to other bacterial diseases that were, prior to this NDM-1 enzyme discovery, so easily cured in the past using antibiotics – then this must surely mean that modern medicine will soon have no sufficient defense against many trivial as well as serious bacterial problems – even against the simplest of bacterial diseases, which must finally result in a huge and sudden rise in morbidity and mortality rates from bacterial infections.

To understand the full import of what I'm saying above, just imagine a world in the future where there are no antibiotics that are effective against C. diff, MRSA, MDR-TB etc. Then imagine no antibiotic cure for the simpler bacterial diseases like UTI infections, kidney infections, E. coli, Klebsiella pneumoneae, Gonorrhea, Salmonella etc. Such will be the effect of the newly discovered NDM-1 enzyme as it continues to spread widely through different bacterial species as predicted. That is, if modern research continues to merely rely on antibiotics against bacterial diseases. Using antibiotics in such a fashion and under such compromised circumstances is like firing expensive blanks at a very dangerous, life-threatening and unstoppable enemy. In the UK

Guardian newspaper, the article describing this phenomenon was titled: *Antibiotic Resistance: Bacteria are Winning the War.*[56,57]

Dimorphism: The Yeast/Fungus Syndrome

I've visited and read many blogs and websites of the so-called experts on candida and many of these experts still persistently refer to candida as just a yeast. This implies the involvement of a singular type of unchanging organism with respect to candida and is therefore highly misleading for the candida sufferer wanting the correct answers to his or her candida problems. Candida is an organism with a dual form. This is well known and accepted through research,[40] and this dual form capability is described as pleomorphic or polymorphic, which means that candida can exist in more than one different structural, functional, behavioral and locational form.[36,37] A bacteria, virus or pathogen that only has one form is called monomorphic. So you can more or less regard a candida infection as eventually evolving and developing into two different and distinct dimorphic organisms that happily coexist— both a yeast form and a fungal form (also called the mycelial form). Both these candida forms are dangerous and debilitating for the body. The purpose of this small section in the book is therefore both to highlight and quickly show you these two forms of candida and to explain the differences between them.

> *"Large fungal forms are present at the end-stages of cancer and AIDS. It is recognised that frequently the cause of death is due to systemic fungus infestations or mycoses. Conventional theory assumes that these are secondary to tumours or the AIDS virus, while the observed pleomorphic life cycle shows that these and their fungal stages are the primary cause why people die of cancer and probably AIDS. The reason for the lethal effects of severe mycoses is probably a combination of poisoning of the energy-producing mitochondria inside cells by fungal toxins and the destruction of erythrocytes by pleomorphics."*
> —*Walter Last (Pleomorphic Microbes)*

There are over 170 different Candida subspecies, only 20 of which are capable of inhabiting the human body because most strains of candida cannot exist in temperatures above 37°C. Candida is certainly confusing because some strains reproduce sexually while others reproduce asexually. Some strains have hypha and others have pseudohyphae and some reproduce using pseudohyphae and budding whereas other candida strains can reproduce using spores. The differences between the dimorphic yeast form and fungal form of candida are quickly summarized below.

* **Structural** – The yeast form consists of ovoid cells that branch into delicate and fragile pseudohyphae. The fungal form has proper robust hyphae that are capable of drilling into host cells to feed as well as to dump their cytoplasm as a defence when under attack. The branching fungal hyphae are also capable of drilling through and damaging the intestinal walls, creating holes in the human intestines that are big enough to allow partially digested proteins to pass through into the blood during digestion. From this leakage, allergies and food sensitivities arise due to these proteins leaked into the blood that are regarded as enemy foreign protein bodies by the immune system, which attacks and removes them—thus causing inflammatory allergic reactions.

* **Nutrition and Feeding** – The yeast form feeds off dead organic matter—a saprophytic feeder. The fungal form is a proper parasite.

* **Behavioural** – The genetic morphing of candida into yeast or fungal forms is entirely governed by the host's body state and where the candida happens to be located in or on the body at the time. If its surrounding host environment consists mostly of dead organic matter (e.g. intestines, skin, mucus), then it will adopt the yeast form, which is as a saprophytic feeder. But if candida finds itself in a host region where there is little or no dead organic matter, then it will adapt and necessarily morph into the fungal, parasitic form and feed directly off the host cells and host nutrients. Both the fungal and the yeast forms excrete poisonous waste into the blood and can happily co-exist in the same environment (e.g. the intestines, uterus etc.).

* Reproduction – In general, the yeast form reproduces and spreads by local budding and the production of local and delicate pseudohyphae, which are always attached to the parent; whereas the fungal or mycelial form reproduces through its more robust and stronger hyphae. In this way, and after using its hypha to drill through the intestinal walls, the fungal form is easily able to disperse and deploy itself more widely throughout the human body using fungal spores.

There are over 20 species of Candida that can infect humans, and the most well known is Candida albicans.

Here is a smaller list of Candida species that are most commonly found to infect humans:

• Candida albicans
• Candida tropicalis
• Candida glabrata
• Candida parapsilosis
• Candida krusei
• Candida lusitaniae
• Candida kefyr
• Candida guilliermondii
• Candida dubliniensis

For the purposes of this book and to avoid any confusion, candida will simply be referred to as Candida albicans or just as candida throughout.

Candida and Biofilms

According to the prolific research, candida biofilm formation is one of the prime reasons why it is so hard to kill and remove candida from the body, and it is perhaps also the most cogent reason why candida keeps returning. Similarly, protective biofilms are also formed by bacterial plaque in the mouth, which is what makes it so hard to kill and remove the bacteria causing gingivitis and gum disease.

Candida biofilms can form in the upper intestines as well as in many other mucus sites in the body. In healthy intestines, a protective mucosal lining forms an alkaline absorption barrier (with an alkaline pH of approx. 8.5) as protection for the inner intestinal villi. When candida infects the upper intestines, it forms biofilms throughout the intestinal mucosa. The waste products exuded from the candida thus create an opposing, poisonous, acid environment while heavy metals in the typically poor human diet are also used and incorporated into the matrices of these complex mucosal biofilms. Biofilms, therefore, not only help to protect the candida and allow it to hide safely from the immune system and from anti-fungal attack, but biofilms will also aid in poisoning the whole body with candida toxic waste, also causing acidosis in the intestines and in the body as well.[41-52]

The latest research has disturbingly revealed that mixed-species pathogens – involving bacteria, viruses and mycoplasma – are able to actually share these candida biofilms, which affords these pathogens additional protection against eradication.[53-55]

The widespread formation of candida biofilms in the body must therefore be regarded as one of the major reasons that regular drug anti-fungals and anti-biotics fail to kill candida and associated bacterial pathogens.[23] As well, despite the huge body of evidence on candida biofilms, I have seen very few anti-candida remedies or protocols that ever even bother to specifically incorporate safe natural surfactants that will actively and swiftly disperse these candida biofilms in order to more effectively expose and kill all the pathogens involved.[24]

Mycotoxicity: The Aldehyde/Alcohol Connection

Now we turn our attention to one of the prime reasons for some of candida's stranger symptoms as exampled by lethargy, brain fog, unclear thinking, mood problems, depression, aches and pains in the body tissues and joints, allergies and sensitivities, deteriorating immune function, weakened liver and low energy levels. Orian Truss first put forward the Aldehyde/Alcohol Connection in his research article, *The*

Acetaldehyde Hypothesis (1984), and more recent research by Weis and Atkins et al. has ultimately proved this theory to be correct.[8,9,10]

These major candida symptoms are all caused when large amounts of aldehydes, alcohols and poisonous proteins are exuded as waste products by the candida into the intestines and into the blood whenever candida infests the body. The liver is the main organ responsible for removing these poisonous substances from the blood, but continual release of these poisonous proteins, aldehydes and alcohols will only ever act to further stress and weaken the liver, hormonal systems and immune system. If these candida waste poisons are not neutralized and quickly removed from the body, then their steady accumulation will systemically weaken the immune system, thereby increasing candida's perpetual dominance in a continual downward health spiral to such an extent until the body's condition becomes chronic, acute or even critical.

The removal of these dangerous candida waste products will be more fully explained and described in the Anti-Candida Strategies Explained chapter.

The Mucus Gland Connection

Normally, entry and infection by candida and other pathogenic infections occurs via the mucus gland sites in the body. These mucus gland sites are found in the following regions of the body:

• Skin
• Nose
• Ears
• Eyes
• Throat
• Lungs
• Stomach
• Uterus
• Intestines
• Breasts
• Prostate

The external mucus glands (consisting of all the above mucus glands with the exception of the prostate and breasts) may be regarded as the human body's first essential line of defense against all incoming pathogens.

I have already made clear the point that candida infections can arise from dysbiosis or from a poor diet. What can also aid in both the infection and rapid spread of candida is an already weakened, immuno-compromised or susceptible immune system. For this to be fully understood and made clear, I will need to quickly describe how the mucus glands normally aid in the defense of the body from outside pathogen attack.

Among the main defensive mechanisms throughout the body are the immune system phagocytes, which act to engulf and continually destroy invasive pathogens. These mucus glands also have two forms of such leukocytes – neutrophils and eosinophils – that help protect against extraneous pathogen attack.

The defensive action against pathogens by both the neutrophils and eosinophils is quite similar. The neutrophils use the myeloperoxidase enzyme (MP) and the eosinophils use the eosinophil peroxidase enzyme (EP) to mediate in the destruction of pathogens such as candida, viruses and bacteria. For ease of understanding, I will only describe how the neutrophil reacts against and kills pathogens.

From a tactile trigger within the mucus, the neutrophil or phagocyte first detects the foreign protein of the pathogen (from bacteria, candida virus etc.) and this stimulates the instantaneous generation of what's called a "respiratory burst" from the neutrophil. This "respiratory burst" comprises a rapid intake of oxygen by the phagocyte, wherein the inner cell conversion of chlorides and iodides occurs and whereby hypoiodous acid (HIO) and hypochlorous acid (HOCl) are formed outside the phagocyte cell via catalysis by the MP enzyme, which mediates this conversion using hydrogen peroxide. The final event of this "respiratory burst" from the neutrophil results in HOCl, HIO and hydrogen peroxide being sprayed outside the neutrophil cell itself. This instantaneously acts to disrupt the outer cell wall of the offending pathogen, resulting in its quick destruction and absorption by the phagocyte. Also a notable feature is that hydrogen peroxide, hypochlorous acid and hypoiodous acid all have distinct pro-oxidant action and are regarded as highly reactive oxygen species. After this event, these pro-oxidants are safely mopped up and removed by anti-oxidants such as catalase and superoxide dismutase. From the research, it has also been found that hypoiodous acid is seven times more efficient at killing pathogens than hypochlorous acid. And in the presence of hydrogen peroxide and either potassium iodide or sodium chloride, purified human myeloperoxidase was rapidly lethal to several species of candida.[84]

Furthermore, the mechanism involved in transferring the iodide to the phagocytes within the blood is wholly reliant on both iodide in the blood and on the de-iodination of the T3 and T4 thyroid hormones—or transfer of iodide from T3 or T4 to the phagocyte cell itself. Therefore if your body is already lacking in proper daily amounts of iodine/iodide – with lowered amounts of thyroxine (T4) and T3 (triiodothyronine) in the blood as a result – then the neutrophil phagocytes will always lack the necessary ammunition in the form of hypoiodous acid to fight pathogens. Hence an inevitable weakening of the immune system occurs due to a lack of iodine/iodide supply and infections and illness increase or are much more pervasive and frequent in the body. (See all the research by *Klebanoff, Lehrer, Stolc and Miller*[84]).

From this critical neutrophil pro-oxidant defense, it therefore becomes much more obvious why supplementing iodine/iodide together with chlorides and hydrogen peroxide is so important for the body. To be more clear, neutrophils store vitamin C for later conversion to hydrogen peroxide. So from the above description, we can safely conclude that iodine, chlorides and vitamin C – in their correct orthomolecular daily amounts – are absolutely essential for a strong immune defense within the mucus glands. Phagocytes in the blood and throughout the body also use this vital standard method of pro-oxidant defense against pathogens in all other regions of the body. So the demand for iodine, chlorides and vitamin C within the body must therefore be quite large. Vitamin C, chlorides and iodine may therefore be thought of as the "ammunition" that the phagocytes urgently require for effective anti-pathogen defence within the body.

Two-time Nobel prizewinner Linus Pauling, from his own research with vitamin C, concluded that people needed to take gram amounts of vitamin C every day—not milligram amounts as recommended by the current RDA. Linus Pauling also concluded that most humans were heavily deficient in vitamin C. With such a deficiency, the majority of humans will therefore have a lack of hydrogen peroxide supply necessary for a healthy immune system.

The immune system's need for sufficient chlorides, as illustrated in the above neutrophil example, is also fairly obvious. Sea salt (unrefined salt) and/or magnesium chloride would seem to be the best supplemental forms for the body to maintain proper chloride levels.

Finally, Dr David Brownstein from the Iodine Utilization Project discovered, through a random trial where he tested 500 people for correct iodine levels by using his Iodine Loading Test, that 94.7% of the people tested were heavily deficient in proper orthomolecular levels of iodine.83 It is perhaps a little easier now to understand how this widespread iodine deficiency might also be significantly contributing to a candida pandemic through a much weakened immune system, which has been caused by a massive lack of iodide/iodine within the Western processed food diet.

From all the above evidence, it is also my own belief that a lack of proper orthomolecular dosages of iodine/iodide, vitamin C and chlorides within the Western diet perhaps constitutes the greatest contributory threat for our immune systems. This is perhaps also a major reason for the explosion of candida problems (as well as many other autoimmune and idiopathic problems) in the Western world in recent years. Please see the following diagram.

Relationship Between Candida, The Mucus Glands and Iodine

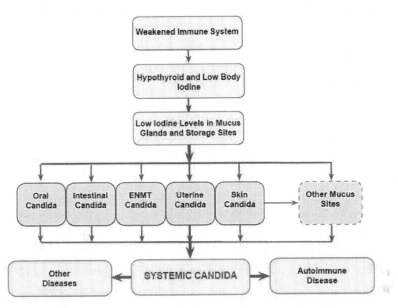

The Hypothyroid Connection

In my own case of systemic candida, I had no doubt at all that I was also low thyroid (hypothyroid) as well because when I first started to take higher doses of Lugol's Iodine it made such a huge difference. Not only did supplementing orthomolecular doses of Lugol's Iodine help to kill pathogens including candida and help to remove heavy metals and halides (bromine and fluorine) from my body, but also my heart arrhythmia and dizziness stopped; I had more energy all of a sudden, clearer thinking; I slept better and all my mucus congestion problems reduced to zero. Furthermore, I am also convinced that iodine helped me to lose excess weight. I have since found out through all the research that supplementing larger dose iodine also has the benefit of making both metabolism and hormonal activity much more efficient. Correct orthomolecular amounts of iodide/iodine are crucial for both the transport and efficient metabolism of fats and proteins in the body, so if you are hypothyroid and these metabolic mechanisms are inefficient then fats will always tend to be stored excessively and you will steadily put on weight, which is what happened in my case.

Needless to say that correct orthomolecular levels of iodine are also needed for the whole body's requirement for iodine and not just required for the thyroid alone. If you are hypothyroid then your immune system's ability to protect your body against any pathogen attack will be greatly diminished. Iodine is part of the essential ammunition that your immune system needs to fight and destroy pathogens.

> *The main causes of suppressed thyroid functions are Candida, mercury and fluoride. Until the 1970's fluoride was prescribed by doctors as thyroid-suppressing medication for patients with an over-active thyroid!*
> *—Walter Last*

To further confuse the issue between candida symptoms and low thyroid or hypothyroid symptoms, both these problems can contribute to causing brain fog, low energy, lethargy, insomnia etc. for different reasons. This can be confusing for not only the ordinary sufferer but can also be confusing for doctors. So if you suspect that you have candida, then you should also get your thyroid levels checked just to be sure. You should avoid the TSH test that doctors usually recommend and insist on having your T3 (triiodothyronine) and T4 (thyroxine) levels checked instead—because this is a much more accurate test. If you have low energy caused by stress issues then it would, perhaps, be advisable to have your adrenals checked as well.

Unfortunately, since this is a book primarily about candida, it is not within its scope to thoroughly cover these hormonal issues in any detail. But if you suspect hypothyroid and/or hypo-adrenal problems associated with your candida issues, then there are some very useful books that have been written that use a more successful and natural approach. Dr David Brownstein, a well known naturopathic doctor, has written a wonderful series of books on both supplementing iodine and on using natural bio-identical hormones instead of synthetic hormones for thyroid and adrenal problems.

Useful books by Dr Brownstein:

Overcoming Thyroid Disorders

The Miracle of Natural Hormones

The Allergy Connection

Another indication of candida is the sudden onset of allergies.[30] This occurs mainly because of the fungal form of candida residing in the gut, where it has the capability to penetrate the intestinal cell wall via the hypha (fungal form). This damage allows partially digested proteins to leak out into the blood from the intestines. These leaked proteins are referred to as foreign protein bodies and are not recognized as friendly host proteins but are, instead, regarded as the enemy by the body's immune system. As a consequence, these leaked proteins are attacked and removed by the white blood cells concurrent with a large release of histamines, resulting in inflammation, discomfort and pain. This problem is also often referred to as Leaky Gut.

Another reason for allergies arising in the body is because of certain other bacterial infections within the gut, such as active mycoplasma, that are also capable of destroying the microscopic finger-like villi and hair-like microvilli of the inner intestinal wall and thus the gut lining. In the intestines, mycoplasma (a fungus-like bacterium) also has known associations with a large number of auto-immune conditions.

The normally advised method for getting rid of allergies is by supplementing large daily amounts of pre-biotics such as lactobacillus or bifido bacteria together with good quality plant-derived protease enzymes containing bromelain and papain. An elimination diet excluding all foods that cause your own allergy reactions must also be followed. In order to heal the intestinal damage, a full course of supportive vitamins and minerals should be included as well. Unfortunately this protocol that I have just described, although very useful for healing the intestines, will not work very well on its own because it is incomplete. If, as I have already made clear, these allergies are indeed caused by candida as well as by other bacterial pathogens, then providing friendly lactobacillus and bifido bacteria will probably not be enough because certain key questions remain unanswered. This regimen will certainly help to make the intestines healthy again—but will it kill the fungal or disseminated candida form (and other bacterial co-infections) that may have already spread from the intestines into the blood? In other words, do pre-biotics act to kill bacteria and fungi already infecting the blood, tissues and organs? No they don't, is the answer. Pre-biotics and pro-biotics will only have beneficial action within the intestines. As I have already mentioned, candida and other bacteria may well be the root cause of allergies, so common sense would seem to dictate that you will not get rid of your allergies for good – with no return of allergies – unless you take the proper and appropriate steps to completely eliminate candida and all pathogen co-infections *from all areas of your body* (not just the intestines) in order to avoid re-infection and return of the allergy problem.

The Autism, ADH, Fibromyalgia, CFS and Alzheimer's Connection

Recent research by Dr William Shaw at his Great Plains Research Laboratories in Kansas has provided several breakthrough discoveries concerning various diseases and several specific metabolic waste products from candida. His research on two specific waste products in particular – tartaric acid and arabinose – seems to provide a definite causative connection between candida and other diseases like autism, Alzheimer's disease, ADHD, fibromyalgia and Chronic Fatigue Syndrome (CFS). In fact, Dr Shaw has been using anti-fungal candida treatments with major success against these and many other difficult diseases.

Tartaric acid is produced in large amounts by candida in the body. Tartaric acid is also poisonous for the body – only requiring 12 gms for it to be lethal. According to Dr Shaw, young autistic children have been found to have high amounts of tartaric acid in their bodies—up to 4.5 gms. Furthermore, tartaric acid is not naturally produced anywhere in the human body, so this acid must only come from a candida yeast infection as the source. Tartaric acid also inhibits or blocks the use of malic acid in the body's citric acid energy cycle, causing hypoglycaemia, and so when tartaric acid gets into the cells and tissues, it can also cause muscle weakness and pain or myalgias. And if, by the same process, the brain does not get enough energy then tiredness, brain fog and lethargy can result—hence the link between candida waste products and other diseases like autism, fibromyalgia, ADHD and CFS.

> *Elevation of yeast metabolites... are found in many of the same disorders and are even more common in autism, SLE, Alzheimer's disease, fibromyalgia, attention deficit hyperactivity, and chronic fatigue syndrome.*
> *—Dr William Shaw*

Arabinose is an aldehyde sugar that is also produced as another waste product by candida. Arabinose is dangerous for the body because it sets up abnormal protein-sugar cross-linking between itself and amino acids such as arginine and lysine to produce a substance called pentosidine. Pentosidine has been found within the characteristic brain tangles of both autistic children and in the brains of people with Alzheimer's disease. It is also believed that pentosidine in these brain tangles contributes to mental problems such as slow thinking, tiredness, brain fog etc. that characteristically occurs in diseases like autism, ADHD and Alzheimer's disease.

The gist of Dr Shaw's research is that it appears to be highly beneficial to use anti-fungals in order to eradicate candida as a major causative factor for these other diseases, thereby eliminating all candida mycotoxins from the body including tartaric acid and arabinose.

Dr Shaw has established links to candida and bacterial toxins in numerous diseases:

• Autism
• Attention Deficit Disorder
• Rett's Syndrome

- Ulcerative Colitis
- Seizures
- Depression
- Child Psychosis
- Fibromyalgia
- Chronic Fatigue Syndrome
- Pervasive Developmental Disorder
- Colitis
- Schizophrenia
- Migraine Headaches
- Alzheimer's Disease
- Systemic Lupus Erythematosus
- Obsessive Compulsive Disorder
- Tourette's Syndrome

(Data Source: Yeast Problems and Bacterial Byproducts)

Dr Peta Cohen,[135] who runs the Total Life Health Center in New Jersey, has also separately confirmed Dr Shaw's research findings. Her approach was to use protease enzymes (nattokinase and lumbrokinase) together with all-natural anti-microbials and anti-fungals, including a heavy metal detox program, in order to eliminate bad bacteria and candida (thereby completely eliminating candida mycotoxins and bacterial toxins from the body). The protease enzyme protocol is used to more rapidly digest and dissolve fibrin-constructed biofilms in the intestines from both fungal and bacterial origin. Removing these biofilms in this way completely de-cloaks the candida and bacteria so that the anti-microbials can more quickly and efficiently kill and remove these offending pathogens.

The results from Dr Cohen's program also confirm that her protocols greatly improve the condition of people with autism, ADH, CFS and fibromylagia problems.

The Dangers of Candida/Bacterial Associations

Several years ago, I advised a woman living in Africa in order to help her to resolve her systemic candida and all her other problems. The total sum of her symptoms, as determined by her doctor from various medical tests, were as follows:

- Candida
- Esophagitis
- Gastritis
- Hiatal Hernia
- Hypothyroid
- Thyroid Nodules
- Uterine Fibroids
- GERD Problems
- Insomnia
- Rapid Weight Loss (28 lbs.)

I immediately advised her to start *The Main Anti-Candida Protocol* along with an extra protocol that would help to cure her GERD problems (supplementing betaine hydrochloride and protease enzymes at mealtimes). However, we had some unfortunate delays of about a month and a half before she was able to get most of the main nutrients (which were somewhat modified due to poor availability of nutrients in her area). She sent me her daily protocol, which is briefly shown here for interest and which I have edited for clarity:

7.00 am: Apple cider vinegar (ACV), water and sodium bicarbonate drink [Alkalizing]

8.00 am: Breakfast [plantains, broccoli, 2 boiled eggs], 2 chanca piedra tablets, 2 desiccated liver tablets, 1 betaine hydrochloride 300mg, 1 vitamin B50 complex, I spirulina tablet 750mg, chlorella tablet 520mg, 1 tablespoon virgin coconut oil (VCO), 1 tablet digestive enzyme or pancreatin, 1 selenium 200ug

9.00 am: Drink borax water, 8 drops of a Fulvic/Humic acid + concentrated alkaline minerals supplement

10.00 am: 8 drops Lugol's Iodine in a glass of water

11.00 am: 1 magnesium citrate 400 mgs, 1000 mgs Lysine, 1000 mgs glutamine

11.30 am: Drink borax in water

12.00 am - 1.00 pm: Lunch [plantains, bit of mashed potatoes or brown rice, chicken or fish, cauliflower or broccoli, greens], 2 chanca piedra tablets, 2 desiccated liver tablets, 1 betaine hydrochloride tablet, 1 tablespoon VCO, 1 tablet digestive enzymes

2.00 pm: Drink borax water, 8 drops of a fulvic/humic acid + concentrated alkaline minerals supplement

3.00 pm: 8 drops Lugol's Iodine in water

4.00 pm: 1 magnesium citrate, 1000mg lysine, 1000 mg glutamine

5.00 pm: Drink borax water

6.00 pm: Omelette fried with VCO

7.30 pm: ACV, water and sodium bicarbonate drink [Alkalizing]

8.30 pm: Dinner [plantains, chicken, broccoli], 2 chanca piedra tablets, 2 liver tablets, 1 betaine HCl tablet, 1 Tablespoon VCO, 1 digestive enzyme tablet, 1 selenium tablet

9.00 pm: 8 drops Lugol's Iodine with water

10.00 pm: 1 magnesium citrate tablet, 1000mg lysine, 1000 mg
glutamine

11.00 or 12 midnight: Bed

This woman followed this protocol religiously every day without fail.
I should also mention that, at the time, she had quite a stressful job
working in a telephone resource centre.

After six months on the above protocol she sent me an email that
simply said she had had a check-up and that she was now in "perfect
health" with all the above symptoms/problems gone.

The reason I've described this testimonial was simply to illustrate the
extent to which other problems or co-infections can occur by association
when you have candida. Notably, all her other problems were also
cured using *The Main Anti-Candida Protocol* (necessarily modified and
adjusted) given in this book, together with a special diet. It's worth
noting that she also supplemented a high daily dose of Lugol's Iodine
– 24 drops of 5% Lugol's Iodine per day (equating to 150 mgs Iodine/
Iodide per day) – with few problems. I have also helped a Filipino and
a man in Indonesia who both had candida problems and they each
took over 30 drops of Lugol's Iodine per day – their own choice – in
their protocols with no adverse side-effects.

From another point of view, candida itself can also regularly be
associated as a co-infection in immuno-compromised patients who
have cancer, HIV/AIDS and other serious auto-immune diseases like
leukemia and hepatitis C.[20] When candida also becomes associated
with these serious disease conditions as a co-infection, as frequently
happens, then the medical situation notably degenerates rapidly,
necessarily becoming much more severe and, if not successfully
resolved, usually results in out-of-control catabolic body degeneration
(body wasting) leading to increased mortality rates.[21,25,27]

Candida Progression in the Body

In its initial form as a yeast, a candida infection may go unnoticed by the sufferer for many years. From this initial infection point, candida has a hold on your body and can spread either rapidly or slowly depending on the candida sufferer's health state at the time, which is so heavily dependent on lifestyle and diet. Candida can also be triggered into its most virulent systemic and fungal form by any number of factors. In my own case, in 2002, I had several candida symptoms that I mistakenly put down to old age (I was 56 at the time). Then, after deciding to retire to the Philippines in 2006, I had eight vaccinations against various tropical diseases as advised by my doctor. I had these eight shots all on the same day and all at the same time. Big mistake! These vaccines, due to their mercury and other toxic contents, were what weakened my immune system giving candida its great opportunity.

Shortly afterwards (after I had moved to the Philippines) two things happened: four of my teeth became loose and just fell out for no good reason and my candida symptoms became greatly exacerbated. In effect, my candida had rapidly morphed into the more virulent fungal form and had invaded my blood, tissues and organs. As a consequence, I started to feel tired all the time; I had brain fog every day and put on weight; I had heart arrhythmia, bad constipation etc. That's when I knew I had candida for sure and that's when I started using the remedies that I now set down in this book. Not only did the candida remedies defeat and remove the candida, but my teeth also stopped falling out and became healthy and strong again.

Please see the following diagram for a greater understanding of how candida can progress and affect the body.

Candida Progression in the Body

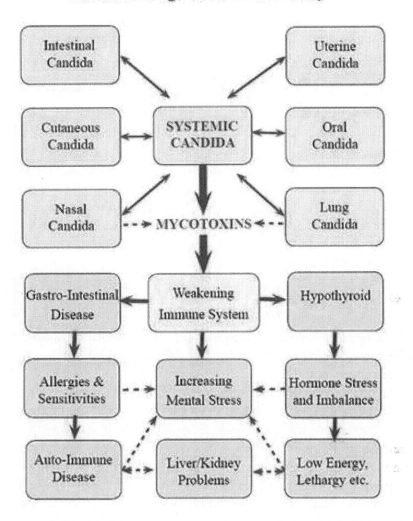

End-Stage Candida Disease

Dr Orian Truss described his first encounter with systemic candida as a young intern during his rounds in an Alabama hospital in 1953, in his book *The Missing Diagnosis*. The patient in question had serious systemic candida. He was severely emaciated in appearance and quite obviously dying. Truss became intrigued with this man's problem so he asked him why he had originally come to the hospital. The patient, a local Alabama farmer, said that he had cut his finger six months previously on his farm and that he had seen his doctor who had recommended antibiotics to stop any further infections. From this point onwards the patient's condition had simply deteriorated over six months into the final catabolic or body wasting stage of systemic candida just before death. The hospital specialists were all completely in the dark as to the reasons why this patient was dying. So Truss decided to put the patient on a larger dose Lugol's Iodine treatment. From that point onwards, the patient started to improve rapidly and within six weeks the man was fully recovered from his severe and chronic candidemia problem.

Characteristically, such as in all serious end-stage autoimmune diseases like cancer, leukemia, hepatitis C or diabetes, catabolic wasting is the body's last desperate and final-ditch attempt to keep the body alive. This destructive catabolic condition is usually characterized by extreme body acidity, eventually giving rise to the metabolic failure of one or more organ systems in the body. The body's various homeostatic mechanisms meanwhile try desperately to counteract and cope with the rapidly building unnatural acidity in the body by robbing amino acids (proteins) from the muscles, tissues and organs and stealing calcium from the bones. Both the ammonia and the calcium derived from these sources help to alkalize the acidity in the body but also tend to create their own significant health problems. Catabolic body wasting – the body visually shrinking in size over a short period of time with sudden and rapid weight loss – is the result of the body trying desperately to survive by cannibalizing itself. All reserves of energy are thus simultaneously depleted, accompanied by inevitable metabolic system or organ failure, as the illness continues to increasingly dominate until coma and, finally, death.

Candida also creates and increases body acidity because of the great amount of acidic poisons (mycotoxins and aflatoxins) released as waste by the candida into the blood. Excess acidity in the body radically interferes with nutrient absorption pathways, excretory pathways, hormones and general metabolism—causing poor energy utilization, underperforming organs and reduced hormonal activity accompanied by a continuously weakening immune system. If the systemic candida infection is not resolved and these poisons and acidity are not simultaneously adequately neutralized and sufficiently removed, then the body will reach an extreme point of acidity, thus triggering the destructive and distinctive catabolic response in the body as its last defense. With no other options left, the body is finally forced to cannibalize itself to survive.

Sheer common sense would suggest that alkalizing the body and neutralizing dangerous acidic build-up is important and highly beneficial as an anti-candida strategy in order to prevent, counteract and halt this body wasting stage. Alkalizing the body neutralizes the excessive levels of acids in the body as well as helping to neutralize and safely remove the offending poisons. For clarification, please see the diagram below.

Like Dr Truss, I have also helped to advise many individuals who were at the more serious catabolic body-wasting stage of candida. In all such cases, I used *The Main Anti-Candida Protocol* shown in this book. The worst candida problem I have ever dealt with was a Filipino man who was working aboard a ship in the merchant marine in Jamaica when he first contacted me for help. This Filipino man was very scared because he really thought that he was dying. Eventually he had to fly back to the Philippines because of his dangerously weakened health state. He told me that when he flew back to Manila, his parents were there to meet him and when his father first caught sight of him, he simply broke down and couldn't stop crying. His son was like a stick insect whose skin had turned completely white (Filipino skin is usually a healthy dark brown). This Filipino man immediately went onto *The Main Anti-Candida Protocol*.

Only one month after he had returned and started the anti-candida protocol, I arranged to meet this man in a hotel. I wanted to know how he was and he wanted to meet me and thank me for my help. To be honest, I really didn't know what to expect. Would he still be emaciated? Would his skin still be white?

I needn't have worried. When he strode into the hotel cafe and extended his hand with a big smile on his face, he appeared as healthy as can be. His eyes were lively and white (not yellow) so his liver was good. His tongue was pink. He was a little on the thin side but by no means skeletal. His handshake was strong and not weak. And his skin was, once again, a healthy dark brown. We spent the whole afternoon walking and visiting places in the area and he did not get tired. He had lots of energy. All good, though I can't take all the credit, as I'm sure that his mother's home cooking played no small part in his recovery as well (his diet was very bad aboard ship).

End-Stage Candida Progression

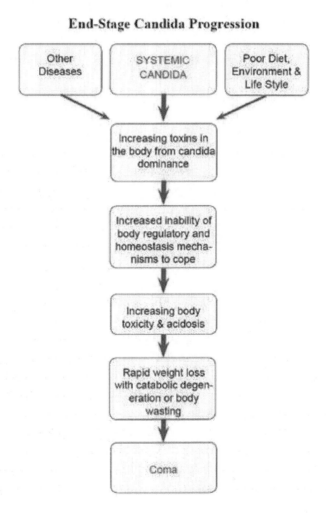

Diet and Intestinal Health

I have come to the conclusion that the intestinal health of our populations has greatly suffered and degenerated as a result of nutritionally poor processed food diets, polluted drinking water and drugs in particular. For instance, many people still earnestly believe that both processed polyunsaturated vegetable oils and refined sugars – in any daily amount – are necessary as a benefit for heart health and energy in particular.

Some years ago I read an interesting article that contained an interview with an esteemed American gastroenterological surgeon. There was nothing particularly revealing or remarkable about this interview until the interviewer eventually asked about his work as a gastroenterologist. The surgeon then happened to mention that, in all his thirty-five or so years as a gastro surgeon, wherein he had operated upon hundreds of patients, he had never actually seen what he would describe as a healthy set of intestines. He then described that the inner lining of healthy intestines should be pink and velvet-like due to the small finger-like villi projecting inwards from the intestinal walls. Instead, the surgeon said that virtually all the intestines he had seen were of a grey appearance, rather like a smooth grey varnish upon the inner lining of the intestines. When the interviewer asked him what he thought the cause was, the surgeon replied, without any hesitation at all, that excessive intake of processed vegetable oils in our diets was undoubtedly the cause.

In 1962, Denham Harman, a much respected English researcher and Nobel Prize winner for his work on the nature of anti-oxidants, undertook a famous experiment. He fed one group of mice their natural diet and he fed the other group of mice the same natural diet together with chemically processed vegetable oil (rapeseed oil). At the end of the experiment he found that the mouse group that had been fed the vegetable oil had a 45% higher rate of cancer than the other mouse group. This was also around the time of Ancel Keys' conflicting research concerning the so-called dangers of eating saturated fats as a specific reason for higher cholesterol levels and heart disease. This research was the basis for belief in the current Lipid Theory on cholesterol and heart disease and was the main driving reason why most people, since the early 1970s, have now switched from saturated fats to using vegetable oils so heavily in their modern diets. Well, here we are some 40 years later and, despite everyone switching to processed vegetable oils in their diet (instead of saturated fats), diseases and problems like high cholesterol levels, high blood pressure and heart disease are nevertheless still logarithmically increasing. So who is right and who is wrong?

In 1995, there was a major research study in South Korea where various body parameters were measured in the national population. There were 2.3 million people who participated in this study, which took place over a 10-year period ending in 2005. Of this number of people being monitored in the study, approximately 20,000 people contracted various types of cancers and underwent the usual allopathic forms of treatment. From the measured parameters, it was found that in all cases of eventual cancer death, the fasting blood glucose levels were above 110 mgs/dL. Of the 3% that actually managed to survive their cancers, all had a fasting blood glucose level of only 90 mgs/dL or below. The lesson to understand here is that excess sugar in the diet helps to promote the growth and spread of cancers. Similarly, it is also important to understand that candida, which is a sugar-loving pathogen, will also grow and spread whenever excess sugars and carbohydrates are eaten in the diet.

My own simpler view and solution is just to follow a *natural diet*. By this I mean a diet that my genes have been naturally used to and expecting for thousands of years. As an example, up until the end of the 1800s the standard fats in our Western diets consisted mainly of tallow, lard and butter—all saturated fats. Similarly during this time period, daily sugar intake was far less than it is today. So, you could perhaps surmise that this type of diet was what our genes were expecting and what they were used to in the diet. Very little vegetable oil and refined sugars were ever deliberately consumed in such large quantities during this earlier period. And as a result of this older diet, there were far fewer occurrences of chronic diseases like heart disease, cancer, Alzheimer's, Parkinson's, diabetes, arteriosclerosis, arthritis, obesity etc. as are so evident today. All because of eating a more natural, higher quality diet. I personally have no problems with vegetable oils as long as these oils are fresh (not oxidized), organic, naturally processed and eaten in the correct smaller amounts that are healthy for the body. For myself, I now only ever use virgin coconut oil – a saturated fat oil – for all my cooking. Saturated fats are more heat stable and are not so easily oxidized. Vegetable oils are polyunsaturated oils, which means that these oils are less stable and more easily oxidized to dangerous trans fats. Thus even organic vegetable oils, as polyunsaturated fats, are in my own opinion not to be trusted because they can so easily be oxidized both in the sunlight and at high cooking temperatures.

There are many items in our modern diets that can wreck your intestinal health. Excessive amounts of refined sugars or carbohydrates, vegetable oils, aspartame, refined salt, drugs, MSG, chemical agri-poisons, a plethora of chemical food additives and preservatives and polluted tap water are just a few examples. The effects of perpetually eating such a poor and acidic diet must therefore surely be sufficient evidence why the vast majority of us do not have pink and healthy intestines.

Summary

Some years ago, perhaps like you, I suffered from the systemic or fungal form of candida and managed to cure this problem myself using the natural remedies recommended by Ted from Bangkok, a resident health expert on the Earth Clinic website. Since that time all those years ago, I have studied and researched candida quite thoroughly in my own way. The major problem inherent in the modern medical approach to candida problems seems to be that after adhering to the allopathic forms of treatment—the candida just keeps returning.[16] So here is a quick reminder of some of the key points and of the fallacies that always seem to prevail concerning candida treatments:

* **Use of antibiotics** against candida will only ever tend to cause dysbiosis and aid the rapid spread of candida, making your problem much worse. See Candida and the Antibiotic Syndrome.[58] Antibiotics

use is one of the top causative reasons for candida infection, persistence and virulence.

* **"Candida is just a yeast."** Not strictly true—it is a half-truth at best. Candida is well known to be dimorphic. It can exist in two different states as two different organisms with completely differing structural, locational, functional and behavioural characteristics. The yeast form is a saprophyte that only feeds off dead organic matter. Consequently, this form resides mainly in areas such as the intestines, skin or uterus of the host. The fungal or mycelial form is a true parasite that feeds more directly off the host itself, with completely differing feeding habits where it also can live and grow in any internal region of the body, including the blood, tissues and organs (including the brain) of the body. This research fact will also help to disprove many of the other fallacies that I'm about to mention concerning candida. The dimorphism or dual form aspect of candida also makes candida a much more difficult organism to defeat – because you are not just dealing with one singular organism but two very different pathogen forms – so common sense would necessarily dictate that your anti-candida strategy should incorporate the appropriate protocols in order to eradicate both the yeast and fungal forms of candida.

* **"If I can get rid of the candida in my intestines then I will be cured."** This kind of thinking is also very wrong. If candida is dimorphic and if its fungal or disseminated form can exist and spread happily into other internal regions of the body besides the intestines, then even if you manage to get rid of the yeast form in the intestines for a while the fungal form in other parts of your body (that you have not killed) will just re-infect and spread back into the intestines. Hence you will have made very little progress in curing your candida—which just keeps returning. This means that in any cure to get rid of candida you will have to target both the yeast and fungal forms. If you don't do this, the candida will just keep returning.

* **"No matter what I try topically to cure my own localized uterine candida problem, it always comes back again."** I have read this so many times in health blogs! This again is bad thinking

and a weak cure strategy that completely forgets or ignores the fact that candida is a dimorphic organism. So if topical remedies for uterine candida or fungal skin problems or fungal sinus problems or localized ENMT candida problems are not working, then **isn't it reasonable to conclude that the localized candida problems (that keep returning) may more realistically be caused by the disseminated or fungal form inside your body and that these localized expressions of candida are merely direct symptoms of a deeper, internal and body-wide systemic candida infection?** So the topical, localized cure strategy will never work and your localized candida problem will keep coming back again and again—this is why you must first cure the internal systemic candida problem to stand any chance of curing your persistent localized candida problem.

* **"All I have to do is just cure my candida, right?"** This is also a bad approach. There are two entirely different dimorphic forms of candida – the yeast and fungal form – that happily coexist and which have completely different locational, structural and behavioural characteristics. It's relatively easy to get rid of just the yeast form in the intestines or locally for a while, but very difficult indeed to get rid of the fungal or systemic form because this form infects everywhere in the body—in the blood, organs and tissues. And if you've had candida for years then it is much more likely that you already have the fungal or systemic form. Add to this that there are a plethora of other pathogens that are usually associated with candida as co-infections, and so this can make candida a very difficult pathogen to both recognize and overcome.

* **Candida has the ability to hide in its own self-created biofilms** and is able to easily avoid anti-fungals and the body's immune defences in this manner. What's more, candida is well known to have myriad associations with other diseases like IBS, Crohn's Disease, Colitis, Leaky Gut, Lyme Disease, Bacterial Vaginitis, Fibromyalgia, Morgellons Disease etc. In one piece of research, cancer sufferers were examined by autopsy to see what the percentage of candida infections were in those who had just died from cancer. They found that 80% of all the cadavers examined had candida. This research was also later separately

verified by other independent research. Similar results were apparent with people who had fibromyalgia—80% of the people examined had candida. The situation is much the same for other end-stage diseases like HIV/AIDS and Hepatitis C where contracting candida as a co-infection can become critically life-threatening. The reasons for these myriad pathogenic associations with candida would seem to be because candida can so easily arise from dysbiosis in the intestines due to antibiotics over-use or anti-immune chemotherapy strategies. Candida is also very effective at further weakening the immune system's defences so that other pathogen species are normally involved within the candida problem as well. The fact that candida is able to shelter itself in biofilms makes candida, with all its apparent pathogenic and parasitic associations, extremely hard to defeat.

* New research has also revealed that mixed-species pathogens – including bacteria, viruses, mycoplasma etc. – also have the ability to share and hide within candida biofilms. This surprising but critically important fact greatly increases the ability of both candida and the other mixed-species pathogens (as co-infections) to resist and survive anti-fungals and anti-microbials, which greatly inhibits their riddance and any eventual cure.

* A long-term bad diet. Like it or not, when people ask the inevitable question on why or how they got candida in the first place – and they can't get rid of it – the answer has to be because of the nutrient-poor processed food diet that person has been eating for the last few decades. A bad diet (bad eating habits in other words) is also a huge factor that helps to both promote and aggravate candida infections. See the Chapter on *The Health Defence Diet* for explanations.

* Other factors. Taking drugs such as steroids, chemotherapy, chemical contraception, anti-depressants and other anti-immune drugs will always act to weaken the immune system to promote candida infections.

CHAPTER 2

Anti-Candida Strategies Explained

In this section, all the nutrients which are used in the anti-candida strategies will be described individually and in summary detail. The succeeding chapter will describe actual details of *The Main Anti-Candida Protocol*, in terms of dosages that can be used. I've separated this information for ease of reference and clarity.

The purpose of this chapter is really to first declare the strategy we will be using against candida. The rest of the chapter will then be devoted to a thorough and fairly detailed description of the nutrients used in all the protocols described in this book.

The anti-candida protocols used in this book comprise the following principles and strategies:

* **Avoid using antibiotics.** Antibiotics are one of the top causes of dysbiosis in the human body—a malady well known to encourage the persistence and spread of candida as well as aiding in and supporting the spread of numerous pathogen problems throughout the body.[58]

* **Directly attacking, killing and removing candida and all co-infections in the body.** These anti-pathogen protocols should be selected and employed to act as wide-acting pathogen killers – that can kill fungi, bacteria, viruses and mycoplasma quickly – while at the same time acting throughout all regions of the body (not just acting in the intestines) for a fuller effect in order to eradicate both the fungal and yeast forms of candida as well as to efficiently kill all the associated pathogens that may also be involved.

* **Removal of heavy metals, halides and other poisons that have accumulated in the body over time.** Apart from greatly depressing and weakening the immune system and liver, heavy metals are a part of

the building material that candida uses to construct biofilms. So heavy metals removal from the body will also help to expose candida and other pathogens by reducing biofilm formation that would normally help to protect and hide various pathogens – including candida – from the body's immune system.

* Using other protocols on a daily basis with specific surfactant or digestive properties that effectively act to dissolve and dispel the biofilms in which candida and other pathogens can protect themselves. By doing this, the involved pathogens will be completely flushed out with nowhere to hide. The candida and pathogen attack remedies can then be more effectively employed to kill and remove the offending pathogens more quickly.

* Alkalizing the body on a daily basis to neutralize bodily acidity caused by anaerobic pathogens, including candida. This also helps to remove toxins, which helps to resolve malabsorption issues in the body. Alkalizing also disrupts biofilms, helps to kill candida, oxygenates the cells, counteracts acidosis and does a myriad other beneficial jobs besides that will be later described.[119]

* Specifically targeting, neutralizing and removing candida mycotoxins and aflatoxins in the body on a daily basis within the protocol. In the 1980s, Orion Truss identified [79] mycotoxins as dangerous waste products from candida. Many of these dangerous candida mycotoxins are also carcinogenic, the accumulated presence of which in the human body is extremely debilitating for the candida sufferer both mentally and physically and which, as a consequence, tends to greatly lower the immune system's effectiveness.[9]

* Strongly supporting the nutritional and excretory pathways of the body – viz. the intestines, liver and kidneys – to help in reducing the inevitable detox and candida die-off or Herxheimer effects so that the blood is quickly purified and healthy again. This is why a simple but wide-ranging liver support protocol is also included in the main candida protocol.

* Supporting and strengthening the immune system and body terrain with vitamin and mineral nutrients that are always lacking in the Western processed food diet. Candida hates a healthy alkaline body with a fully functioning and strong immune system.

* Strictly following an Anti-Candida Diet – Follow the Health Defence Diet.

So from above and in a nutshell, any anti-candida protocol that you adopt must comprise and fulfill the following strategy criteria to successfully and completely eradicate systemic candida and all associated pathogenic co-infections:

Anti-Candida and Anti-Pathogen Protocols

Anti-Biofilm Protocols

Alkalizing Protocols

Essential Detox Protocols

Liver Support Protocols

Vitamin and Mineral Support (Immune System Support)

The Health Defence Diet

Candida Attack Protocols

The candida attack protocols are an essential part of removing candida from the body and comprise the following protocols:
• Lugol's Iodine
• Borax or Sodium Tetraborate
• Alkalizing
• Pau D'Arco
• Methylene Blue

Candida sufferers should also choose and use at least three of the candida kill protocols from the above list. I make no secret that my own favourite threesome is to use Lugol's Iodine, borax and the alkalizing protocols. Some therefore might wonder why I even bother to give more candida attack protocol options. I've helped candida sufferers in Asia, the Middle East and in Africa and, in many instances, people in these regions are simply unable to purchase Lugol's Iodine or borax because they are either unobtainable or because of the expense. That is why I also include other options in the above list.

Lugol's Iodine

Lugol's Iodine (LI) is also known as Aqueous Iodine (UK) and comprises a mixture of water, 10% potassium iodide and 5% molecular iodine together in solution. Since its discovery and formulation by Jean Lugol in 1829, Lugol's Iodine has had a long and useful history in medicine with an almost unparalleled ability to quickly kill different forms of pathogen species.

As an example of this pathogen-killing capability, please see the figure below.

Speed of Kill of PVD Iodine Against Bacteria, Yeast/Fungus and Parasites

ORGANISMS (Number of Strains)	PVP Iodine Used in ppm(range)	KILL TIME In seconds	ORGANISMS (No. of Strains)	PVP Iodine Used in ppm(range)	Kill Time In seconds
Proteus(41)	100 – 2500	15 – 180	Trichophyton(2)	1000	60
Staphylococcus(36)	66 – 2500	15 – 80	Aspergillus(2)	1000	30
Pseudomonas	25 – 2500	15 – 900	Mima(1)	2500	60
Escherichia(23)	200 2500	15 – 30	Herella(1)	2500	60
Salmonella(9)	1000 – 2500	15 – 60	Edwardsiella(1)	2500	60
Candida(8)	3.75 – 2500	10 – 120	Citrobacter(1)	2500	60
Serratia(6)	200 2500	60 – 120	Providencia(1)	1000	60
Spores-Bacillus Clostridium	10000	2 – 5 hrs	Acinetobacter	3.75	10
Trichomonas(5)	400 – 2500	30 – 60	Epidermophyton	1000	60
Enterobacter(4)	1000 – 2500	60	Microsporum(1)	1000	60
Klebsiella(4)	500 - 2500	60	Penicillium(1)	1000	30
Clostridium(4)	1000	30 – 60	Nocardia	2500	60
Shigella(3)	1000 - 2500	60	Sarcinia(2)	500 - 2500	60
Corneybacterium(3)	2500 60 -120	60	Bacillus(3	7.5 - 2500	60
Diplococcus(3)	1000 -2500	60	Mycobacteria(3)	1000 - 2500	60 -120

(Data Source: *Bring Back the Universal Nutrient Medicine.* IMVA article; *http://www.health-science-spirit.com/iodine.html*)

The above table describes the speed-of-kill of povidone iodine (PVD) against several species of bacteria, fungi and parasites whose properties are exactly the same as for Lugol's Iodine. It should also be noted that Lugol's Iodine has equal speed-of-kill efficacy against many viruses.

A quick summary of the beneficial properties of Lugol's Iodine is given below:

- Essential for proper thyroid health.
- Useful anti-oxidant.
- Efficient anti-pathogen—kills most forms of bacteria, viruses and fungi quickly.
- Effectively works to reverse hypo- and hyperthyroid conditions.
- Has anti-biofilm surfactant properties.
- Acts as an anti-histamine at larger dosages.
- Detoxes cadmium, aluminium, lead, mercury, arsenic and other poisons.
- Detoxes fluorine and bromine.
- Helps to balance the body's hormone system.
- Essential for all hormone receptor activity and health (not just the thyroid gland).
- Raises metabolism, making it more efficient.
- Essential for proper immune system health.
- Essential immune system component of mucus glands throughout the body.
- Essential for bone health.
- Promotes skin, hair and nail health.
- Promotes healthy digestion.
- Reduces excessive mucus production.
- Helps regulate estrogen in the ovaries.
- Decreases insulin needs/helps diabetes.
- Iodine has mucolytic action (clears excess mucus in the lungs, nose etc.).
- Increases energy (increases ATP production).
- Essential for early brain development.
- Lowers cholesterol and reduces arterial plaque build-up.
- Radiation protection.

Overcoming Problems Supplementing Lugol's Iodine

In this section I will be addressing several well-known problems that can arise on starting the higher dose Lugol's Iodine protocol. Notably, as I will prove, these problems are not caused by the iodine itself but arise from bad dietary and lifestyle choices.

In helping people with their candida problems in various countries, I have noticed that people in the West, particularly from modern societies who consume processed food every day, have a much greater sensitivity to supplementing Lugol's Iodine (LI). These people seem the most likely to achieve peculiar reactions and sensitivities to LI, which gives rise to symptoms like anxiety, arrhythmia, rashes, hives, insomnia etc. Conversely, whenever I have helped people with candida issues who live in the less developed regions such as in the Philippines, Indonesia or Pakistan, these candida sufferers, as a general rule, do not tend to suffer from any of these peculiar reactions from supplementing larger doses of Lugol's Iodine.

What is the reason for this strange anomaly?

The answer to this question is simply food quality, and by quality I mean food that is grown, raised and eaten in its most natural and healthy state. In this respect and in my own humble opinion, Western processed food has a very low quality score indeed. Western food is grown with a plethora of fertilizers, pesticides, fungicides, drugs and many other unnatural agri-chemicals. Then the food is heavily processed after harvesting or slaughter, using evermore chemicals including chemical preservatives and additives. By contrast, in underdeveloped countries such as Indonesia or the Philippines, it has been my experience that food is normally sold and purchased fresh in the wet markets, with little use of chemical fertilizers or heavy and unnatural chemical processing. As a result, the Western diet inevitably causes the unnatural build-up of heavy metals and halides such as chlorine, fluorine and bromine and many other poisons in the human body over decades; whereas there is much less build-up of these dangerous chemicals in people from underdeveloped countries whose food is more naturally grown and naturally prepared.

Iodine is by far the best antibiotic, antiviral and antiseptic of all time.
–Dr David Derry

Consequently, when a person from the West starts to supplement higher dose Lugol's Iodine for the first time, then most likely he or she will already have a large store of heavy metals and other toxic chemicals in the body. But a person from the Philippines or Indonesia for instance, because they eat more natural foods and much less of chemically prepared foods, will have a much smaller amount of foreign chemicals and poisons already stored in their bodies. As a consequence of this fact, people from these underdeveloped regions seem to have little or no problems supplementing higher doses of Lugol's Iodine.

Iodine is a very efficient detoxer of aluminium, cadmium, lead, mercury and arsenic as well as being an efficient detoxer of fluorine and bromine among many other poisons. So when a person on a lifetime processed food diet, with large amounts of poisons already stored in his or her body, first begins the higher dose iodine protocol, then the stored poisons will suddenly be released in large quantities by the effects of the iodine and dumped into the blood—with all those peculiar symptoms of anxiety, skin rashes, insomnia, arrhythmia, depression etc. occurring due to untold stress on the liver.

Furthermore, it has also been my own observation that people from the more underdeveloped regions of Africa, the Middle East and Asia are easily able to begin a higher dose Lugol's Iodine supplementation without any major issues or problems because their own food supplies are fresher and more naturally prepared without so many fertilizers with unnatural chemical content.

Another problem, which is also linked to this food quality issue, is the apparent lack of beneficial nutrients in our Western processed food. When you begin to supplement higher doses of Lugol's Iodine and you already have a major deficiency in certain essential or critical anti-oxidants in your diet, then it is also possible that iodine supplementation at higher dosages could result in an autoimmune reaction against the thyroid gland with eventual formation of thyroid nodules. I must also quickly add here, before my readers all throw their hands up and scream "Poison!" in unison, that for well over a hundred years, right up until the World War II period, Lugol's Iodine was used heavily by the medical profession at dosages of up to 2000 mgs per day (equivalent to 320 drops of 5% Lugol's Iodine) for a multitude of acute and chronic conditions without causing any major problems or harm. I have even read one piece of historic medical research where doctors used Lugol's Iodine at a dose of 20 grams a day to help successfully cure syphilis. Simply put, Western diets were far healthier up until the World War II period. But shortly after this period, ever-increasing agri-chemical use, chemical food processing and additives, preservatives and GMO really came into their own in the West. As a result, we now have many hidden poisons in our diets as well as a critical lack of nutrients and anti-oxidants in our food supply.[75,76,77]

> *Medical textbooks contain several vital pieces of misinformation about the essential element Iodine, which may have caused more human misery and death than both world wars combined.*
> *–Dr Guy Abraham*

As Dr Guy Abraham from the Iodine Project has so adequately proved from his own historical, medical and demographic research on iodine, the Japanese as a population eat particularly large amounts of seaweed/kelp. Their daily intake of iodine/iodide from this seaweed diet has been calculated from research to be 13.8 mgs per day,[77-79] which is around 80 to 100 times more than the current RDA of 150 micrograms for iodine/iodide. The FDA, however, still today maintains that taking more than 1 to 2 mgs of iodine/iodide per day acts to poison the thyroid despite all the common sense evidence, convincing historic proof and sensible arguments to the contrary. The FDA's current judgment and recommendations upon supplementing iodine is wholly based on one particularly weak piece of research by Wolff-Chaikoff in 1948. Dr Guy Abraham successfully rebutted the findings of the *Wolff/Chaikoff Report* in his own research paper: *The Wolff-Chaikoff Effect: Crying Wolf?*[74]

Furthermore, within his own more recent research, Dr Guy Abraham has already completely explained the biochemical reasons for thyroid nodule formation whenever higher dose iodine is supplemented. Within the thyroid cell itself, thyroglobulin is normally converted to T3 (triiodothyronine) and T4 (thyroxine) via moderation by the thyroid peroxidase catalytic enzyme. This conversion process quite naturally produces hydrogen peroxide as a normal byproduct of reaction. But if glutathione peroxidase – a critical enzyme and anti-oxidant for the thyroid – is not present in the thyroid cell in appropriate amounts, then a dangerous build-up of hydrogen peroxide will occur within the thyroid cell itself. Excess hydrogen peroxide build-up further acts to change the nature of the thyroid peroxidase protein so that the immune system is unable to recognize it anymore as friendly host protein. As a consequence, the antibodies will attack and remove this "foreign" thyroid peroxidase enzyme so essential for T3 and T4 production in the body. The excess hydrogen peroxide builds up to unhealthy levels, which also tends to disrupt and destroy thyroid cells, with resulting thyroid nodule formation.[81]

> *Iodine is needed in microgram amounts for the thyroid, mg amounts for breast and other tissues, and can be used therapeutically in gram amounts.*
> *–Dr. Donald Miller Jr.*

In order to avoid this thyroid nodule problem caused by a lack of glutathione peroxidase whenever higher dose Lugol's Iodine is supplemented, the following companion nutrients should always be supplemented at proper orthomolecular dosages: vitamin C, magnesium, selenium, B50 complex and higher dose niacin.[82,83] These iodine companion nutrients, which are all usually depleted or missing in our processed food diets anyway, assure correct body amounts of glutathione peroxidase and other essential minerals while providing anti-oxidants that are critical to the production of thyroid hormones without problems. These iodine companion nutrients are all incorporated within *The Main Anti-Candida Protocol* in this book.

So again I'll say it as a reminder. These thyroid problems are not actually caused by the Lugol's Iodine itself. These problems must, instead, be due to our poor quality Western food diets that are so laden with dangerous toxic chemicals and so heavily lacking in important nutrients and critically supportive anti-oxidants.

For myself, I have been taking 8 drops or 50 mgs 5% Lugol's Iodine for the last six years on a daily basis and I have never had any problems with the higher dosage. I take all the iodine companion nutrients mentioned above as well. The most noticeable immediate effect of supplementing with higher doses of Lugol's Iodine is a clear mind and greater energy levels. The most noticeable long-term effect has been cleared mucus in the chest and in the nose (iodine has mucolytic action) and I have not caught a cold or flu or any infectious disease for the last six or seven years since starting to supplement daily iodine in this manner.

> *Iodine is utilized by every hormone receptor in the body. The absence of iodine causes a hormonal dysfunction that can be seen with practically every hormone inside the body.*
> *–Dr George Flechas*

For more extensive details and evidence on the medical history, demographic use, safety and proper supplementation of iodine at orthomolecular dosages, see the Resource Index for more details.[74-81]

Other useful and relevant book resources:

- *Iodine: Why You Need It, Why You Can't Live Without It* by Dr David Brownstein.

- *The Missing Diagnosis* by Dr Orian Truss.

Borax Water

Borax is another essential part of the anti-candida protocol because it is, perhaps, the ultimate fungal killer. Borax, or sodium tetraborate, also kills other pathogenic bacteria such as mycoplasma and helps to both alkalize and remove fluorine from the body. Borax aids in properly regulating bone formation and helps to balance the body's hormones. Furthermore, according to the Material Safety Data Sheet on borax (MSDS is the bible for researching toxicity), borax has about the same toxicity level as common table salt.

Rex Newham, a demographic biological researcher also discovered that supplementing borax cures arthritis (i.e. that borax or boron deficiency can cause arthritis). Rex Newham, at the age of 33, had severe arthritis in his hands but he managed to completely cure his own arthritis in only a few months by just supplementing borax.[96] His useful and honest research on borax and arthritis in the 1970s has been completely and deliberately ignored by medical research. See the article, *The Borax Conspiracy*, by Walter Last[94] for more details.

Ted from Bangkok recommends supplementing borax water for candida and for other problems such as arthritis, ticks and mite problems. The way you make the borax water is simply to add 1/8 teaspoon of borax to one litre of mineral water. The protocol simply involves drinking a litre of the borax water every day on a five days on, two days off basis. Borax is a strong anti-fungal and as such an essential ingredient in *The Main Anti-Candida Protocol*.

Alkalizing

Very few, if any, alkalizing protocols are used in any of the other anti-candida remedies that I have read about on the internet. Alkalizing the body on a daily basis – using Ted from Bangkok's alkalizing remedies from EarthClinic.com – is one of the healthiest protocols you can use because these protocols strongly rebalance the body's health. It helps the body's homeostasis mechanism and electrochemistry bring certain body parameters – such as pH, conductivity and redox potential – back to healthy levels again.

Some of the benefits of alkalizing the body are listed below:

- Improves chelation and promotes removal of heavy metals from the body
- Increases the oxygenation of the body
- Creates a bad environment for pathogens
- Reduces tissue pain by reducing acidity
- Reduces general pain by neutralizing lactic acid—a major cause of pain
- Reduces constipation caused by acidity
- Reduces diarrhea caused by excess body acidity
- Healthy blood pressure depends on proper nitric oxide levels, acidity destroys it
- Blood vessel constriction causes high blood pressure if the body is too acid
- Excess arterial clogging due to acidity causes strokes
- Excess acidity (below pH 6) causes kidney dysfunctions and damage
- Sports fatigue is due to acidity build-up in the body
- Recovery from strokes is dependent on achieving proper body alkalinity
- Free radicals build-up occurs as acidity levels increase
- Glycation, glaucoma, and cataracts increase as body acidity increases
- Virus, fungus and other pathogen communities proliferate in the body when body pH is too acid
- Pancreas function depends on bicarbonates, without which pancreatic beta cells get destroyed
- Improves malabsorption issues in the body
- Helps to remove toxins
- Improves digestion
- Helps to oxygenate the body
- Helps to prevent mutation abnormalities in the body's DNA
- Improves body energy
- Improves blood circulation
- Improves the electrochemical activity or conductivity of the body
- Improves the redox potential of the body—making the body less oxidative
- Improves and supports the immune system
- Improves and supports body homeostasis

There are three simple remedies that can be used for alkalizing the body on a daily basis.

1. Sodium Bicarbonate and Water – Alkalizing the Blood
This remedy is highly useful for alkalizing the intestines and the blood. Baking soda (sodium bicarbonate) has been used for over a hundred years as a household cleaner to kill mold and fungus.

2. Lemon/Lime, Baking Soda and Water – Alkalizing the Cells
This protocol is specifically used for intracellular alkalization, which also helps to increase energy levels via the citric acid cycle in the body.

3. Apple Cider Vinegar, Baking Soda and Water
This remedy can be taken as an alternative to the Lemon/Lime and Baking Soda remedy. This also alkalizes the intracellular environment and helps to increase body energy due to its malate and acetate content.

For a better understanding on this complex subject and more in-depth information on alkalizing the body, you can either visit the *EarthClinic. com* website (See Ted's Alkalizing Formulas) or refer to the ebook called *pH Balanced for Life: The Easiest Way to Alkalize* by Parhatsathid Napatalung (aka Ted from Bangkok) and Bill Thompson.

Pau D'Arco
Pau D'Arco is a well known Amazon rainforest tree with many medicinal actions: antifungal, anti-bacterial, antiviral, kills leukemia cells, relieves pain, reduces inflammation, fights free radicals, reduces tumours, enhances immunity, thins blood, relieves rheumatism, reduces mucus and secretions.

Pau D'Arco is also used widely throughout the native tribes of South America against malaria, anaemia, colitis, respiratory problems, colds, cough, flu, fungal infections, fever, arthritis and rheumatism, snakebite, poor circulation, boils, syphilis, and cancer.

Normally supplemented as a bark decoction, tea or as a tincture. Capsules/tablets are not advised.

(Source: Raintree Tropical Plant Database; *http://www.rain-tree.com/paudarco.htm#.UgUaU2RoRKU*)

Methylene Blue

The proper chemical name for Methylene Blue (MB) is methylthioninium chloride. Methylene Blue was discovered in 1891 by Paul Ehrlich and has the following beneficial properties: anti-fungal, anti-bacterial, anti-parasitic, anti-protozoal, methylating agent (increases energy). It is used in aquaculture to kill fungi, protozoa and bacteria.

This anti-fungal remedy is normally supplemented as drops in a glass containing vitamin C as ascorbate dissolved in water. Taking Methylene Blue in this way will prevent the side-effects of blue whites of the eyes and green urine. This remedy should not be taken after 3 pm due to its stimulating and energizing methylation effects on the body, which may prevent sleep in the evening if taken after this time.

Anti-Biofilm Protocols

The anti-biofilm protocols that are employed in *The Main Anti-Candida Protocol* are necessary and essential to remove any safe hiding place for the candida. Not addressing and removing biofilms is usually one of the major reasons why candida sufferers fail with their own protocols and is one of the key reasons why candida keeps returning. If you don't specifically act to sufficiently inhibit, dispel or destroy candida biofilms, then candida will be easily able to avoid any anti-fungal that you are supplementing.

Examples of nutrients used in *The Main Anti-Candida Protocol* that help to destroy biofilms or inhibit their formation are given here:

Turpentine/Kerosene
Protease Enzyme Protocol
Lugol's Iodine
Humic Acid
Borax
Alkalizing

Since the majority of the above remedies have already been described, I will only describe the action of the Turpentine/Kerosene Protocol and the Protease Enzyme Protocol in detail—because these two modalities are also the strongest and most efficient protocols for getting rid of mature, hardened biofilms.

The two anti-biofilm protocols shown below should only be used if there is little or no progress with the normal protocols given in this book. In such cases it is normally the case that hardened biofilm formations in the intestines are what mainly inhibit the protocol's success. Therefore in such instances, where a mature biofilm has had the chance to form over a longer period of time, stronger anti-biofilm protocols must necessarily be used.

One of the greatest reasons for the failure of any anti-candida protocol is the lack of any specifically active or useful anti-biofilm components within the protocol itself, which leads to inadequate removal of biofilms from the gut and body resulting in candida return and persistence.

When candida infests the intestines it hides in the mucus layers and more or less takes over this region. In the later more serious stages, after the candida has spread body-wide, the nutritional pathways will also be hugely compromised by the candida, partially due to biofilm formation. So the main reason that the candida-kill remedies may not be working so well is most probably due to the wide extent of protective candida biofilm formation in the gut/body. These biofilms are where the candida and other bacteria hide, where they can successfully avoid anti-fungals or antibiotics and where they can so easily evade the immune system.[41-52]

Over time and at a later stage, these immature biofilm micro-slime formations eventually become hardened, mature biofilms (the same as bacterial plaque on teeth – also made from biofilms) thus becoming much more difficult to dislodge and disperse. So you will need to supplement stronger anti-biofilm nutrients to dislodge, dissolve and dispel the biofilms in order to fully expose the candida so that the anti-fungals – such as iodine, borax, humic acid, molybdenum, alkalizing etc. – are able to actually reach and kill the candida itself. Therefore, you must take stronger anti-biofilm nutrients to more efficiently expose the candida in your body.

When these biofilms are rapidly dispersed, there is also a large accompanied release of heavy metals in the intestines (heavy metals are always used in biofilm formation), which could be re-absorbed back into the body via the colon. So it is also advisable to supplement chlorella, sodium thiosulfate and other heavy metal detoxifiers when you undergo this protocol.

When biofilms initially form, they are an immature liquid micro-slime. Within the biofilms themselves, pathogens – including candida – can fulfill all their metabolic functions while at the same time being fully protected within the biofilm layer itself. And as time passes, the biofilm layers become hardened and even more difficult to remove.

This is when you should, perhaps, consider using the Turpentine/Kerosene Protocol or the Protease Enzyme Protocol because both these modalities remove biofilms quickly.

The Turpentine/Kerosene Protocol

You can use either turpentine or kerosene for your protocols because they are very similar in chemical composition. Turpentine, derived from the distilled gum sap of pine trees, is the stronger version being higher in beneficial pinenes and terpenoids than kerosene. Therefore turpentine is generally taken a teaspoon at a time, whereas kerosene can be taken at higher dosages. To complicate matters further, kerosene is also called paraffin in the UK and in some other parts of the world. Furthermore, some paraffin – such as Pink Paraffin or Blue Paraffin – should **not** be used in this protocol because of unhelpful additives.

Finally, the reason turpentine or kerosene is such an efficient anti-candida remedy is because it both kills candida quickly and also removes candida biofilms very rapidly. Both kerosene and turpentine are used as a paint thinner and as a paint stripper, so these surfactant properties make kerosene or turpentine uniquely ideal for rapidly removing candida biofilms.

Turpentine, or gum oil of pines, is derived directly from the distilled sap of pine tree bark, whereas kerosene is mainly derived from distilled coal or petroleum products (which also come from the geothermal breakdown, over time, of plants and trees within the rock strata). Only distilled low odour forms of turpentine or kerosene should be used, with a boiling point range of between about 150°C - 200°C.

From this point on, for ease of description, I will be referring to kerosene/turpentine as pine oil or turpentine. The health benefits of just the *alpha-pinene* and *beta-pinene* content of turpentine are listed below:

Alpha-Pinenes
• Lipophilic
• Bactericidal
• Fungicidal
• Insecticidal
• Pesticidal
• Anticarcinogenic (cytotoxic on cancer cells)
• Diuretic
• Antioxidant
• Immunostimulant
• Anti-inflammatory
• Anti-convulsive
• Sedative
• Anti-stress
• Hypoglycaemic
• Capable of expelling xenobiotics (substances, such as drugs, poisons and toxins, which are foreign to the human body)
• Anticholinesterase activity (prevents destruction of neurotransmitters in the body)

Beta-Pinenes

- Lipophilic
- Bactericidal
- Fungicidal
- Insecticidal
- Acting against osteoclasts (thus increasing and improving bone formation and bone density)
- Anticarcinogenic (cytotoxic on cancer cells)
- Pesticidal
- Antioxidant
- Sedative

(Data Source: *The Essential Oil of Turpentine and its Major Volatile Fraction (alpha- and beta-pinenes): A Review, http://www.imp.lodz.pl/upload/oficyna/artykuly/pdf/full/--04_09_Mercier.pdf*)

The main reasons that supplementing turpentine rids candida and other pathogens so rapidly from the body is due to its anti-fungal, lipophilic, antibacterial, hypoglycaemic (lowers blood sugar), immuno-stimulant, anti-oxidant and anti-parasitic qualities. And the fact that turpentine is a well-known natural paint stripper simply adds to its rather unique ability to rapidly strip-away and dissolve difficult biofilms.

I even, through my own interest, had a look through the 1899 Merck Manual for medical doctors and I was truly astonished by the extent to which turpentine was medically used in the past for all sorts of problems like respiratory diseases, digestive and intestinal problems, and for even more severe problems like gonorrhoea and syphilis. Notably, as Dr Jennifer Daniels points out in her article *The Candida Cleaner*,[58] the 1999 Merck Manual suddenly declared turpentine to be a dangerous poison despite hundreds of years of useful and successful medical use. There is also further solid historic and testimonial evidence that both turpentine and kerosene have been successfully used to cure many forms of cancers.[85,86,87]

Please also take note that even though the turpentine/kerosene protocol is very simple, it is a very strong and fast-acting remedy against candida. I have read several testimonials where just using the turpentine or kerosene protocol alone has cleared serious candida problems in a matter of a few weeks. But because of its wide, rapid-kill effect on candida and a host of other pathogens and because of its unique ability to clear biofilms and detox the body so quickly, be forewarned that if you supplement turpentine, it is highly likely that you will get a significant Herxheimer (die-off) and detox healing crisis when you initiate this turpentine protocol. That is why you should follow the tenet "start small and go slow"; increase turpentine dosages and frequency slowly to the proper advised daily dose so that your body can get used to the protocol and be able to cope. Dr. Jennifer Daniels also recommends initially taking laxatives and eating a proper healthy diet before you actually start the protocol because of the initial laxative and clearing effects of the turpentine on the body, and I would advise the same. Let me also add that there have never been any recorded instances where the turpentine/kerosene protocol has ever seriously harmed anyone.[90]

There are three ways to undergo the turpentine protocol:

* Taking a teaspoon of turpentine with sugar (as recommended by Dr Jennifer Daniels) just before meals.[88] The turpentine will then be carried into the intestines with the food—mainly helping to rid candida from the intestinal region. This method, as Dr Daniels also relates, served to maintain the good health of plantation slaves in early America. It was their secret cure-all and tonic for all ills.

* Taking a teaspoon of turpentine with a teaspoon of castor oil (or olive oil) mixed with a glass of milk as Walter Last recommends.[89] I tend to favour taking the turpentine with either Virgin Coconut Oil or Black Seed Oil (Nigella sativa) because of the added anti-pathogen and protective healing effects contributed by these carrier oils. This method also carries the turpentine into the intestines to help knock out the candida.

* Taking a teaspoon of turpentine in a glass of water or milk on an empty stomach (outside mealtimes). The stomach rapidly absorbs the

turpentine directly into the blood for best action and effect against the fungal or disseminated candida form that infects the blood, tissues and organs (outside the intestines). This method has been successfully and widely used for all sorts of serious diseases including candida, tuberculosis, polio, cancer, meningitis and leukemia and is still being used in Russia, the Russian satellite countries, Germany, Poland and in Africa to good effect as an effective and cheap remedy and all-around tonic for the body.[86]

For more detailed evidence on the history, safety and use of supplementing turpentine/kerosene please refer to the Resource Index.

The Protease Enzyme Protocol
Protease enzymes digest and dissolve proteins. Candida biofilms – or any biofilms for that matter – start out as micro-slime that initially consists of an immature and weak lattice or matrix structure made of fibrin (think of it as a microscopic fibrin cage within the mucus) that becomes over time a much denser, stronger and harder fibrin mass due to the increased spread of fibrin. This cage or fibrin matrix imparts amazing protection for the candida and other pathogens that are residing in this biofilm matrix. Biofilm matrices are like impenetrable fortresses where neither anti-microbial or anti-fungal supplements nor the immune system is able to reach the pathogens residing safely within.

Fibrin is a form of protein. Therefore using protease enzymes within the protocols acts to completely digest the fibrin, which exposes the candida residing within the biofilm mass so that the anti-fungals and anti-microbial ingredients used in the protocol will much more effectively and quickly be able to kill these offending pathogens.

In her own research, Dr Peta Cohen, founder of the Total Life Center in New Jersey, has also found that removal of biofilms helps to rapidly resolve problems in diseases like autism, chronic fatigue syndrome (CFS) and fibromyalgia (all these diseases are commonly associated with candida).[135-138] In his book, *The Yeast Connection: A Medical Breakthrough*, Dr William Crook likewise confirmed an important connection between such diseases and candida. Additionally, Dr Peta Cohen identified through her own research that biofilms incorporate heavy metals as well as other metals in excess – like iron, calcium and copper – into the fibrin matrices of these biofilms in the intestines. She discovered that when the protease enzymes (such as nattokinase or lumbrokinase) are used in her protocols, large amounts of heavy metals and other metals (incorporated into the fibrin matrix biofilm structure) are suddenly released into the intestines. Therefore it also becomes an imperative to simultaneously neutralize these dangerous released heavy metals using other detox ingredients like EDTA (ethylenediaminetetraacetic acid), chlorella or sodium thiosulfate (see the next section – Essential Detox Protocols) to ensure quick and safe removal in order to prevent re-distribution of these heavy metals throughout the body via their re-absorption in the colon.

Other alternative and much cheaper forms of protease enzyme that you can use in the same way are bromelain and papain. Bromelain and papain are derived from plant protease enzymes, from pineapple and papaya respectively. Their fibrinolytic actions in the intestines are exactly the same as for nattokinase and lumbrokinase. These plant protease enzymes have the added advantage that they will happily work to digest protein – as fibrin – in either an acid or an alkaline medium.[137,138]

For candida sufferers, proteolytic enzymes (nattokinase, lumbrokinase, bromelain and papain) are normally supplemented outside mealtimes so that these enzymes will not act on food but will only act on and remove the fibrin from biofilms in the intestines.

Essential Body Detox

Detoxing is particularly important for successfully removing candida from the body. It is well-known and already fairly well accepted that heavy metals and halides (chlorine, fluorine and bromine) occur as significant content in tap water, drugs and in processed foods today. Such foreign toxins are particularly difficult to remove from the body and, in the case of heavy metals, they usually get stored all over the body within fats. Therefore these candida toxins will steadily accumulate in the body over time, having the effect of upsetting metabolism and greatly lowering the immune system's capabilities, thus giving candida free rein to spread further throughout the body.

Another aspect of heavy metals is that they are normally a requirement and a further boost to the spread of candida because they are always used to help manufacture candida biofilms (See the Anti-Biofilm Protocols section). So by constantly detoxing in your anti-candida protocols, this will also help to remove biofilms from the body. Within the protocols, strong detoxing nutrients such as chlorella, iodine, hydrogen peroxide, alpha lipoic acid, milk thistle, vitamin C, sodium thiosulfate, selenium, cilantro and other supporting anti-oxidant nutrients are also strongly advised as part of the heavy metal detox procedure.

The main nutrients employed in the protocols to remove chlorine, fluorine and bromine are sodium thiosulfate (chlorine removal), Lugol's Iodine (fluorine and bromine removal) and borax (fluorine removal).

Another important but separate part of the detox procedure needed against candida is for the constant neutralization and removal of fungal aflatoxins and mycotoxins – poisonous candida waste products – from the body. These candida toxins, as they continually accumulate, will radically affect metabolic processes making them less efficient. These toxins will also act to greatly upset and stress the body's hormone balance, immune system and liver. Candida waste toxins will therefore act to greatly stress the body over time both physically and mentally in terms of energy loss, giving rise to the more peculiar candida symptoms of brain fog, unclear thinking, lethargy, tiredness, myalgia etc.

In his book, *The Missing Diagnosis,* which was written in the 1980s, Dr Orian Truss identified 79 fungal mycotoxins in candida waste products. That number of discovered candida mycotoxins has increased to over 200 today. He also proposed, in a 1984 research article called *The Aldehyde Hypothesis,*[7] that the large amounts of aldehydes and alcohols excreted by candida as waste products into the blood were responsible for many of the more peculiar and debilitating mental and physical effects of candida as a pathogen. Later on, due to some particularly good research work from Weiss J, Cooter S, Schmidt W, et al., Truss's hypothesis was proved to be correct.[9]

Within the body, human aldehyde dehydrogenase is the main enzyme that neutralizes and clears dangerous excessive aldehydes and alcohols in the blood. The central metallic component of aldehyde dehydrogenase is molybdenum, a very necessary and useful trace element for the human body. Other forms of molybdenum – molybdate and ammonium molybdate in particular – have, for years, been used in agriculture as an additive in small amounts to prevent wheat rust (fungus) occurring in grain stores. So molybdenum has further usefulness because it kills the fungus/yeast as well. The aldehyde dehydrogenase enzyme converts both excess alcohols and aldehydes circulating in the body to acetic acid, which is a particularly useful substance used in the energy pathways and the production of co-enzyme A. So taking molybdenum on a daily basis will also act to kill the candida, helping to reduce and eliminate fungal and yeast mycotoxins as well as helping to increase personal energy levels. Molybdenum is used as a main component in *The Main Anti-Candida Protocol*. Interestingly, use of molybdenum is rarely found in any of the other anti-candida protocols that I have seen.[8,9]

In his book, *The Alpha Lipoic Acid Breakthrough*, Dr Berkson has shown from his own considerable research and experience how the use of his simple *Triple Anti-Oxidant Therapy (Selenium, Milk Thistle and ALA)*, can offer huge protection against fungal aflatoxins, mycotoxins and other toxins in the body. This therapy strongly protects the liver and the excretory pathways and is essential to help purify the blood from toxic waste and other dangerous trash.

Dr Berkson relates in his book how when he was a young intern the hospital specialists had given up on a patient who was badly poisoned by eating poisonous mushrooms. This patient, the medical experts said, was going to die. Not satisfied with this prognosis, Dr Berkson immediately contacted a research friend and asked if there was anything he could try to save his patient. The friend suggested Alpha

Lipoic Acid (ALA) to be given both by IV and orally—this was in the 1970s when very little was known about the health effects of ALA. So his research friend sent him some ALA and Dr Berkson used the suggested protocol on the critically poisoned patient, who recovered to full health in only two weeks, much to the great embarrassment and anger of all the so-called medical specialists at the hospital who thought that recovery was simply not possible.

Liver and Kidney Support

The above section is perhaps reason enough to include ALA, milk thistle and selenium (The Liver and Kidney Support Protocol) in your anti-candida protocols. Both ALA and milk thistle are wonderful detoxifiers, greatly aiding in support of the liver while helping to promote kidney health as well. Selenium is used in the protocol not only as an anti-oxidant and to help detox mercury, but to also help generate glutathione and glutathione peroxidase, two essential anti-oxidants for the body that both help to efficiently remove free radicals and eliminate toxic poisons from the body—thus greatly helping to reduce candida aflatoxins and mycotoxins in the blood while also greatly aiding liver, kidney and thyroid function from the protocol's strong anti-oxidant action.

Vitamin and Mineral Support

I've already mentioned that modern processed food lacks vital minerals and vitamins. So the majority of nutrients advised in this section are required to increase these essential nutrients for the body in order to help strengthen many body health parameters including digestion, enzymes, hormones and the immune system. This part of the protocol also rapidly increases and reinforces the amount of active anti-oxidants in the body, thus raising the body's health state in many ways.

Magnesium: Magnesium is used in over 325 enzyme processes in the body. Magnesium is essential to regulate calcium and to help regulate bone formation. It is essential for thyroid function, digestion and energy as well as for proper central nervous system and immune system function yet is one of the major nutrients lacking in our Western diet today.

Vitamin C: Another primary anti-oxidant vitamin that is hugely lacking in our diets. Vitamin C is essential to the support of the immune system; this vitamin is also needed for collagen cell repair, heavy metal chelation and is essential, in larger and proper orthomolecular amounts, to help prevent disease.

Zinc: Essential for the body, it acts as an anti-oxidant and helps to greatly boost the immune system. Zinc is essential for the production of superoxide dismutase and is also highly beneficial for the intestines. Zinc is involved in the production of over 100 different enzymes in the body and is essential for protecting and repairing cells.

Niacin and the B Vitamins: Essential for the proper functioning of digestion, the central nervous system, energy pathways, digestion and certain hormones. Niacin, at larger orthomolecular dosages, tends to greatly strengthen the immune system, cure depression, lower blood pressure and improves blood transport to the peripherals of the body. The most recent research on vitamin B3 has also discovered that taking niacinamide (non-flush form of B3) will increase the strength of the immune system by a factor of 2000.

Virgin Coconut Oil (VCO): Contains mainly medium chain saturated fatty acids – which are highly protective for the intestines – such as lauric acid, capric acid, caprylic acid, caproic acid and myristic acid. These also act as useful anti-microbials that kill both candida and bacteria in the intestines as well as helping to protect the intestines against any further microbial invasions.

Humic/Fulvic Acid: Antiviral, anti-bacterial and anti-fungal; improves and balances the body's metabolism; chelates heavy metals; alkalizes; provides a huge range of minerals for the body's needs; balances the body's electrochemistry.

Sea Salt: Provides a wide range of minerals for the body; essential for healthy operation of the sodium symporter networks for blood/cell mineral transport and nutrient exchange; necessary for saline balance in the blood; provides essential chlorides for the body to help both the digestive process and to help the immune system.

When people decide to take this simple Vitamin and Mineral Support Protocol, many request if they can just take these minerals and nutrients more conveniently as multivitamins. I am against the use of multivitamins for the following reasons:

• Multivitamins do not contain vitamins, minerals or amino acids in their correct orthomolecular amounts—as advised in the protocol in this book. In general, all dosages within multivitamin tablets are well below even the RDA. If multivitamins actually contained the proper recommended orthomolecular dosages of minerals, vitamins and amino acids required for daily health, then that multivitamin pill should, by rights, be the size of a ping-pong ball.

• As a general rule, multivitamins do not dissolve properly in the intestines because of the way they are made. Therefore they will be useless to you because the body cannot absorb them. If you don't believe me, then drop a hard multivitamin tablet into a glass of water. It should completely dissolve in the glass of water within 15 minutes. If it does not dissolve in this time, then it is useless.

• Multivitamins contain all sorts of unhelpful additives – including wax-like caking agents such as magnesium stearate, stearic acid, calcium diphosphate, starch, cellulose etc. – that actually hinder absorption of nutrients into the body.

• Combining minerals in their inorganic forms such as magnesium, calcium and zinc into a single multivitamin pill is not beneficial because these and other minerals will compete for the same nutritional pathways into the body.

Hard tablet forms are therefore the worst form to use to supplement nutrients for all the above reasons. Pure powder forms or capsules containing powders should always be used instead.

The Health Defence Diet

Any anti-candida protocol worthy of any merit must always include a proper and strict anti-candida diet. A processed food diet will do little to help cure your candida problems. So taking anti-candida remedies without a proper anti-candida diet is like taking two steps forward with your anti-candida protocols and three steps backward because you are still eating processed food that is contaminated with toxins and greatly lacking in proper and essential nutrients.

See Chapter 3 – The Health Defence Diet – for more detailed information.

Summary and Comparisons

Within this chapter, I have tried to explain all the good reasons why you should use all the ingredient's within *The Main Anti-Candida Protocol*. When compared to other anti-candida protocols, these others are generally found to be lacking in certain nutrient strategies that are so essential for successfully resolving candida problems. These other protocols do not consistently work so well because:

• Their strategies are too simplistic and only ever focus on just killing the candida and doing nothing else.

• Some only use Nystatin as the main candida-kill ingredient. It is well known that Nystatin is very poorly absorbed into the body from the intestines[136,137] so it will have little effect in removing the fungal or disseminated candida form that infects the blood, tissues and organs (outside the intestines). As a result of this poor strategy, the candida will just keep returning.

• They permit or rely on antibiotics. Antibiotics act to increase the spread and virulence of candida.

• These other protocols don't overtly use any strong anti-biofilm components in their protocols and that's another reason why the candida just keeps coming back.

• These other protocols do not even attempt to kill or remove any of the associated bacterial co-infections and other problems that are always so intimately involved with candida problems.

• Very few of these other protocols use molybdenum to both neutralize candida mycotoxins and kill candida.

• Very few, if any, of the other protocols that I've read about use Lugol's Iodine, borax or alkalizing as essential components against candida.

The above reasons are what makes *The Main Anti-Candida Protocol* given in this book both completely unique and stronger in approach and much more effective against all forms of serious candida yeast/fungal infections.

Few people perhaps realize how adaptable and robust candida is as a pathogen. The extent to which candida can invade so many different regions in the body is truly surprising. Various forms of candida can invade the following areas of the body: intestines, lungs, bone, joints, skin, nose, eyes, central nervous system, heart, liver, uterus, biliary, spleen, pancreas, peritoneum and bladder.

For a complete index on the extent of how candida yeast/fungus can infect the human body, see the The *DoctorFungus.org* website (The Mycosis Study Group).

CHAPTER 3

The Main Anti-Candida Protocol

This section will be devoted to describing the guidelines for the protocol, showing the necessary dosages and other useful information in note format as well as giving an example of the daily protocols schedule in table format for both simplicity and as a helpful quick reference.

Before you start this protocol, it would also make complete sense to have a hair analysis done in order to determine exactly what heavy metals you have inside your body in excess and also to discover what minerals and vitamins you are lacking from your diet. The hair analysis will ultimately help you to more accurately fine-tune the nutrients that you are taking within this protocol to your individual needs in order to achieve a more accurately balanced and healing protocol.

If you suspect an allergic reaction might occur with any of the ingredients within the protocol, then you should first test for allergy reactions on your skin. To do this, place one drop or a small amount of the suspect nutrient on the skin, in the crook of your arm, and leave it there for several hours. If, at the end of this time, you have redness or itching in that area, then you may well be allergic to that substance; but if there is no redness, itching or irritation then you are most probably not allergic to that substance.

Protocol Guidelines

Candida sufferers should essentially use the following guidelines in their protocols:

• Stop taking antibiotics unless absolutely neccessary. Antibiotics will kill all the beneficial bacteria in the gut and help to create acid intestines and dysbiosis via a condition called the Antibiotic Syndrome. This is highly beneficial to the spread and virulence of candida.

• Always use the Anti-Candida Diet.

• Always use the alkalizing remedies.

• Use at least three of the main candida-attack remedies within your protocol. Lugol's Iodine, borax and alkalizing are my own favourites for killing candida.

• Use vitamins, minerals and herbs in their most natural organic forms wherever possible. Avoid "chemically standardized" herbs. Use the purer powder forms or powder capsules, not hard tablets.

• If any particular nutrient in the protocol is causing problems, then either reduce the dose or pulse the full dose once every three days. Stop supplementing that nutrient if an allergic reaction is confirmed.

• Always use protocols that remove and detox heavy metals, halogens (fluoride, bromide, chorine) and other toxic chemical poisons or mycotoxins from the body. Poisons drag down the body's immune system, acidify the body and create the perfect environment for candida.

• It is strongly advised that all the vitamin and mineral support nutrients are also taken **in their proper orthomolecular amounts as advised.** These nutrients help to address other metabolic problems – such as low immune system, over-stressed liver or low thyroid – that may also contribute to and exacerbate candida problems.

• Liver and kidney anti-oxidant support is also strongly advised in all cases where there is a heavy or severe die-off or detox effect, which tends to stress the liver and kidneys thus causing nausea and flu-like symptoms.

• The Anti-Candida Diet is a no-brainer when you ask yourself, "How did I get candida in the first place?"

If progress and healing or recovery is slow while using these protocols then you should additionally take one of the stronger Anti-Biofilm Protocols—either the Turpentine/Kerosene Protocol or the Protease Enzyme Protocol as described in Chapter 2. Reducing candida biofilms will greatly accelerate recovery and cure.

The Detox or Die-off (Herxheimer Effect) Healing Crisis

It has been my own experience that people will always get an initial die-off reaction of some sort when moving onto an anti-candida protocol such as this one. A die-off or a detox reaction is due to large amounts of candida debris, mycotoxins and/or heavy metals or halogens being released into the blood, which will cause particular stress on the immune system, liver and kidneys. So liver/kidney and immune support and anti-oxidant support are strongly advised to help alleviate the die-off/detox symptoms (this is included in the protocol). A reduction in anti-candida and/or detox dosages may also be required for a while to make the healing crisis more bearable for the user. When people are infected with systemic candida and they attempt a cure, **they should always expect an initial period of time during which they may feel considerably worse due to these die-off and detox reactions. This die-off reaction is actually a good sign and proves that the protocol is working against the candida.** This die-off or Herx or detox reaction will vary from person to person and its duration will depend both on the extent and stage of the candida infection as well as the extent to which the body has stored heavy metals and other poisons. It will also depend on the current health state of the individual at the time. This is a completely normal and medically recognized reaction that will last until the candida debris and poisons are removed from the body. It will also depend on when the immune system once more is able to dominate and control the body's health.

Candida Attack Protocols

Lugol's Iodine

Dosage: 4 drops (25 mgs)

Frequency: Taken 4 times a day (16 drops total)

Total Daily Dosage of Lugol's Iodine: 100 mgs.

Taken outside mealtimes

Work up to the full dosage and frequency slowly

Activity: anti-viral, anti-bacterial, anti-fungal – essential for the thyroid gland – anti-cancer – essential for whole body iodine needs – helps to regulate the body's hormones – reduces mucus – raises metabolic efficiency – increases energy – chelates heavy metals – removes fluorine and bromine from the body – helps regulate proper bone formation – essential as ammunition for the immune system.

Alternatives: All above drop dosages are given assuming 5% Lugol's Iodine strength is being used (6.25 mgs per drop). For other Lugol's Iodine strengths, adjust drop dosages accordingly. See the Lugol's Iodine drop-to-mgs conversion chart below:

Lugol's Iodine Drop to Mgs Conversion Chart

Lugol's Solution Concentration (dosage calculated per drop)	Iodide	Iodine	Total Dosage
2%	1.50 mg	1.0 mg	2.50 mg
3%	2.25 mg	1.5 mg	3.75 mg
5%	3.75 mg	2.5 mg	6.25 mg
7%	5.25 mg	3.5 mg	8.75 mg
10%	7.50 mg	5.0 mg	12.50 mg
15%	11.25 mg	18.75 mg	7.5 mg

(Data Source: *http://www.breastcancerchoices.org/lugolschart.html*)

Source and Availability: Pharmacies, chemists or from internet vendors.

Comment: Make sure to slowly work up to the daily iodine dosage given above. The Iodine Protocol companion nutrients should always also be taken along with Lugol's Iodine supplementation to avoid problems (See Chapter 2 for details). These iodine companion nutrients are already incorporated within both the Vitamin and Mineral Support and Liver and Kidney Support Protocols.

Caveats: None.

Borax Water

1/8 of teaspoon borax

Add to one litre of mineral water

Drink one litre of this solution throughout the day

Take this remedy for 5 days only, then take 2 days off this protocol

Activity: kills yeast/fungus – kills mycoplasma and other bacteria – regulates bone maintenance – insecticidal – helps to regulate the body's hormones – removes fluoride from the body – alkalizes the body.

Alternatives: None.

Source or Availability: 20 Mule Team Borax, internet vendors.

Comment: This protocol should be taken continuously on a 5 days on, 2 days off basis.

Caveats: See the Earth Clinic website for a list of reader reported side effects.

Alkalizing Protocols

Sodium Bicarbonate and Water

1/4 - 1/2 teaspoon of baking soda (sodium bicarbonate)

Add to half glass of water

Frequency: 3 times a day

Supplemented one hour after all meals

Activity: kills yeast/fungus – improves digestion – improves body electrochemistry – improves body pH, Redox Potential and Conductivity – alkalizes the blood.

Alternatives: None.

Source or Availability: Arm & Hammer Baking Soda, Bob's Red Mill Baking Soda, internet vendors.

Comment: Alkalizes the blood.

Caveats: None.

Lemon or Lime and Baking Soda with Water

One squeezed whole lemon or lime

Add 1/4 - 1/2 teaspoon baking soda until the fizzing stops

Mix all in half glass of water

Frequency: 2 or 3 times a day

Taken outside mealtimes

Activity: kills yeast/fungus – alkalizes the intracellular environment – increases energy – improves cellular electrochemistry.

Alternatives: Ted from Bangkok's apple cider vinegar (ACV) with baking soda and water remedy. Two tablespoons of ACV are used per dose— prepared exactly the same as above. See *EarthClinic.com* for details.

Source or Availability: Arm & Hammer Baking Soda, Bob's Red Mill Baking Soda and ACV from supermarkets, health shops and internet vendors.

Comment: Add the baking soda to the lemon/lime and water mixture until the fizzing stops. Alkalizes the intracellular environment. Both the above protocols should be used in the protocols—to alkalize the blood and the cells simultaneously.

Caveats: None.

Methylene Blue

0.1% Methylene Blue (MB) solution is used

Add 1/4 teaspoon vitamin C sodium ascorbate to a glass of water

Add 10 drops 0.1% Methylene Blue (colour will go from blue to clear)

Frequency: Taken twice a day

Second dose should be taken before 3 pm in the afternoon

Activity: kills yeast/fungus, bacteria, plasmodia, trichomonas etc. – increases energy by methylation.

Alternatives: None.

Source or Availability: Aquaculture or aquarium shops. Internet vendors.

Comment: The second MB dose should be taken before 3 pm in the afternoon because Methylene Blue is so energizing and stimulating due to its methylation effects.

Caveats: Must be taken together with vitamin C to avoid whites of the eyes turning blue and green urine side-effects. No such problems occur when taken with orthomolecular dosages of vitamin C. Should not be supplemented at the same time as Lugol's Iodine.

Pau D'Arco

Taken as the organic tincture, decoction or tea forms

Dosage: As recommended

Frequency: 3 or more times per day

Work up to the full dosage/frequency slowly

Activity: strongly anti-fungal – antibacterial, anti-viral – anti-cancer – shrinks tumours – anti-leukemia – relieves pain – kills parasites – thins blood – enhances immunity – relieves rheumatism – removes free-radicals.

Alternatives: Cat's Claw (Uncaria tomentosa).

Source or Availability: Health shops, internet vendors.

Comment: Can create strong Herx or die-off effects. Start small and go slow with the dosage and frequency.

Caveats: No known side-effects.

Anti-Biofilm Protocols

The Turpentine/Kerosene Protocol

There are 3 ways to take this protocol:

1st Method
Dosage: Supplement 1 teaspoon of sugar mixed with 1 teaspoon of turpentine

Frequency: Normally supplemented three times a week or as required

Can be taken with or without food

Work up to the full dosage slowly

2nd Method
Dosage: A glass of milk supplemented with 1 teaspoon of olive oil, castor oil or coconut oil mixed with 1 teaspoon of turpentine

Frequency: Normally supplemented three times a week or as required

Can be taken with or without food

Work up to the full dosage slowly

3rd Method
Dosage: One teaspoon of turpentine in a glass of water

Frequency: Normally supplemented three times a week or as required

Supplemented outside mealtimes for best absorption directly from the stomach into the blood

Work up to the full dosage slowly

Activity: antifungal, anti-bacterial, anti-viral, anti-parasitic – rapidly removes biofilms – cleanses the intestines – pesticidal – insecticidal – anti-worm – anti-oxidant – diuretic – anti-carcinogenic – immunostimulant – anti-inflammatory – anti-convulsive – sedative – anti-stress – hypoglycaemic – removes poisons from the body – promotes bone formation.

Alternatives: Kerosene.

Source or Availability: Hardware/camping shops, internet vendors.

Comment: Health effects are mainly due to alpha- and beta-pinene and limonene content. Can cause strong Detox or Herx die-off effects. Start small and go slow with the dosage and frequency when initially starting this protocol. If stools become too loose or the die-off or detox effect is too severe, reduce frequency and dosages accordingly.

Caveats: Can create laxative effects if the dosage is too large. Adjust dosage and frequency accordingly.

The Protease Enzyme Protocol

Supplement nattokinase or lumbrokinase enzymes

Dosage: As recommended

Frequency: Supplemented at least 3 times a day outside mealtimes

Activity: digests and dissolves biofilms (fibrin) – anti-inflammatory – reduces pain – cleans the blood, removes blockages (dead organic protein) – helps the immune system do its job.

Alternatives: Bromelain and papain plant enzymes are another cheaper option that can be just as effective to use for removing biofilms.

Source or Availability: Health shops, internet vendors.

Comment: Can trigger strong heavy metal detox healing crisis. Because large amounts of heavy metals are also suddenly released from the biofilms, it is therefore important to ensure that heavy metal detox supplements are also taken simultaneously when using this protocol. If stools become too loose or the die-off or detox effect is too severe, cut back on frequency and dosages accordingly.

Caveats: None.

Essential Detox Protocols

Sodium Thiosulfate
10% sodium thiosulfate solution is used

Dosage: 6 to 10 drops of sodium thiosulfate in a glass of water

Frequency: Once a day

Supplemented outside mealtimes

Activity: detoxes heavy metals, arsenic, cyanide and chlorine – kills fungus – anti-oxidant.
Alternatives: None.

Source or Availability: Aquatic or aquarium shops, internet vendors.

Comment: None.

Caveats: Can have a laxative effect when you first begin to supplement sodium thiosulfate.

Chlorella

Dosage: 300 mg to 500 mg

Frequency: 3 times a day

Supplemented at mealtimes

Activity: Detoxes and removes heavy metals from the body.

Alternatives: None.

Source or Availability: Health shops and internet vendors.

Comment: The alginates in chlorella ensure that the heavy metals are expelled quickly from the body without re-absorption or redistribution.

Caveats: Can sometimes create significant detox reactions—adjust dosage/frequency accordingly.

Molybdenum

Molybdenum or sodium molybdate forms are used

Dosage: 900 micrograms

Frequency: 3 times a day

Supplemented outside mealtimes

Activity: removes poisonous alcohols and aldehydes (fungal mycotoxins) from the blood – kills candida.

Alternatives: None.

Source or Availability: Health shops, internet vendors.

Comment: Ted from Bangkok recommends supplementing higher dosages of molybdenum at 10 mg to 25 mg a day for only two weeks. It is difficult to find or purchase molybdenum at dosages higher than 900 mcg (RDA maximum). Sodium molybdate has a low toxicity profile (LD50 of 4gms/kg in rats).

Caveats: None.

Vitamin and Mineral Support

Vitamin C

The sodium ascorbate form should be used (not ascorbic acid)

Dosage: 1000 mgs

Frequency: 3 times a day

Taken outside mealtimes

Activity: major anti-oxidant – essential for collagen repair – chelator of heavy metals – helps prevent arteriosclerosis and heart disease – anti-cancer – strong immune booster.

Alternatives: Magnesium ascorbate (difficult to find).

Source or Availability: Health shops, internet vendors.

Comment: To create your own sodium ascorbate, first make a solution of ascorbic acid in water and add baking soda (sodium bicarbonate) slowly to the solution until the fizzing stops. Now you have sodium ascorbate that you can supplement in solution. Calcium ascorbate should be avoided.

Caveats: None.

Zinc
Dosage: 25 mgs

Frequency: Once a day

Taken with meals or outside mealtimes

Activity: anti-oxidant – immuno-stimulant – helps repair and protect the intestines – regulates proper hormone levels – required for normal libido – anti-stress – benefits the blood, bones, liver, kidneys and retina (eyes).

Alternatives: Zinc citrate, zinc acetate, zinc gluconate.

Source or Availability: Health shops, internet vendors.

Comment: The 25 mg zinc dosage should only be taken for a maximum of two weeks, then the frequency should be changed to 25 mgs once a week, otherwise excess zinc side-effects may occur.

Caveats: None.

Magnesium

Magnesium chloride is the best form to supplement

Dosage: 250 mgs

Frequency: Twice a day

Taken with meals or outside mealtimes

Activity: regulates calcium and bone formation – essential for the thyroid gland – anti-bacterial – immune-booster – protects heart health – protects digestion and the intestines.

Alternatives: Magnesium oil (10 drops per dose), magnesium citrate, magnesium gluconate.

Source or Availability: Health shops, internet vendors.

Comment: Magnesium is an essential part of the anti-candida protocol because most people will be deficient in this mineral.

Caveats: None.

Humic/Fulvic Acid

Taken as the liquid, powder, granule or capsule form

To supplement, the humic/fulvic acid in water should have a light golden colour (not black)

Supplement dosage as recommended

Frequency: As recommended

Activity: cleanses, neutralizes and removes toxins – removes heavy metals from the body – alkalizes – improves and balances metabolism – improves the body's electrochemistry – re-mineralizes – anti-viral, anti-bacterial, anti-fungal – immune booster – oxygenates the blood – improves metabolism – increases energy.

Alternatives: Shilajit capsules (Ayurvedic Medicine).

Source or Availability: Health shops, internet vendors.

Comment: I take the granulated humic/fulvic acid form. All I need for one dose is just three tiny granules added to a glass of water to turn the colour to a light golden brown colour.

Caveats: None.

Virgin Coconut Oil
Only virgin coconut oil (VCO) should be used

Dosage: One tablespoon

Frequency: Twice a day

Supplemented at mealtimes

Activity: antibacterial, anti-fungal, antiviral – protects and supports the intestines – supports the thyroid – reduces adipose tissue (fat) – hepato-protective – anti-inflammatory – analgesic – anti-pyretic (anti-fever).

Alternatives: None.

Source or Availability: Health shops, supermarkets, internet vendors.

Comment: I've been using VCO for all my cooking for the last six years and wouldn't use any other cooking oil now because of all its beneficial effects.

Caveats: None.

Sea Salt
Only sea salt should be used (not refined salt)

Dosage: 1/4 teaspoon

Frequency: Twice a day

Activity: Immune booster – essential for the body's sodium symporter networks (blood/cell mineral exchange) – essential for serum electrolyte balance – essential for stomach acid production – supplies a wide range of trace minerals for the body – regulates heartbeat – regulates and reduces mucus – alkalizes the body.

Alternatives: Rock Salt (natural).

Source or Availability: Health shops, internet vendors.

Comment: None.

Caveats: None.

Niacin
The niacin (causes flush) or niacinamide (non-flush) forms may be used

Dosage: 500 mgs

Frequency: Twice a day

Supplemented with meals

Activity: anti-oxidant – reduces depression, improves mood – lowers cholesterol – increases the strength of the immune system by a factor of 2000 – lowers cholesterol (niacin form only) – anti-oxidant – aids digestion – safely thins the blood (niacin form only) – increases energy.

Alternatives: Niacin or niacinamide.

Source or Availability: Health shops, internet vendors.

Comment: Niacin is the better form to take because it has more beneficial action. To avoid the niacin flush, take an aspirin 20 minutes before you take niacin or take niacin at mealtimes. Niacin should always be taken with all the other B vitamins because the effect is synergistic.

Caveats: None.

B50 Complex

B50 complex should be supplemented

Dosage: As recommended

Frequency: Once a day

Supplemented at mealtimes

Activity: wide ranging benefits for the skin, central nervous system, digestion and energy – immune boosting and hormone balancing – antioxidant – protects the heart – protects DNA – improves memory – regulates blood sugar.

Alternatives: None.

Source or Availability: Health shops, internet vendors.

Comment: We are all lacking in the proper daily amounts of B vitamins due to our poor diets.

Caveats: None.

Liver and Kidney Support Protocols

Alpha Lipoic Acid

The RS or R-ALA forms may be used

Dosage: 300 mgs

Frequency: Twice a day

Supplemented at mealtimes

Activity: removes heavy metals from the body – both oil and water soluble – regenerates used up anti-oxidants in the body – increases energy – removes poisons from the body – aids and protects the liver and kidneys – anti-oxidant – hypoglycaemic – regenerates and repairs nerve tissue – prevents DNA damage to cells – protects heart health – anti-aging.

Alternatives: None.

Source or Availability: Health shops and internet vendors.

Comment: None.

Caveats: None.

Milk Thistle

Dosage: 1000 mgs

Frequency: Supplemented twice a day

Taken at mealtimes

Activity: removes poisons from the body – aids and protects the liver and kidneys – anti-oxidant actions – regenerates and repairs the liver – anti-cancer.

Alternatives: Dandelion root.

Source or Availability: Health shops and internet vendors.

Comment: None.

Caveats: None.

Selenium

Dosage: 200 micrograms

Frequency: Supplemented twice a day

Taken at mealtimes

Activity: immuno-stimulant – anti-cancer – generates glutathione and glutathione peroxidase as essential anti-oxidants – removes mercury from the body – hepatoprotective – protects the thyroid gland – protects the heart.

Alternatives: None.

Source or Availability: Health shops and internet vendors.

Comment: None.

Caveats: None.

Example Daily Protocol Schedules

Morning Protocol Schedule

Time	Meal	Supplement	Amount/Dose	Comment
7:00 am		Sea Salt	1/4 tspn	Taken with water.
8:00 am	Breakfast	Magnesium Zinc B50 Complex Niacin Chlorella	250 mgs 25 mgs As recommended 500 mgs As recommended	Taken with water.
9:00 am		Sodium Bicarbonate	1/4 to 1/2 tspn	Taken in 1/2 glass of water.
10:00 am		Molybdenum	900 mcgs	Taken with water.
11:00 am		5% Lugol's Iodine Lemon or Lime Juice and Baking Soda Vitamin C Powder Humic/Fulvic Acid	4 drops One whole lemon/lime 1/4 to 1/2 tspn 1000 mgs As recommended	All taken together mixed with water.
12:00		Molybdenum	900 mcgs	Taken with water.

Afternoon/Evening Protocol Schedule

Time	Meal	Supplement	Amount/Dose	Comment
1:00 pm	Lunch	Alpha Lipoic Acid Selenium Milk Thistle Niacin Chlorella Coconut Oil	300 mgs 200 mcgs 900 - 1000 mgs 500 mgs As recommended One Tablespoon	Taken with water.
2:00 pm		Sodium Bicarbonate Sea Salt	1/4 to 1/2 tspn 1/4 tspn	All taken mixed with water.
3:00 pm		5% Lugol's Iodine Lemon or Lime Juice and Baking Soda Vitamin C Powder	4 drops One whole lemon/lime 1/4 to 1/2 tspn 1000 mgs	All taken together in a glass of water.
4:00 pm		Molybdenum	900 mcgs	Taken with water.
5:00 pm	Dinner	Magnesium Alpha Lipoic Acid Selenium Milk Thistle Chlorella Coconut Oil	250 mgs 300 mgs 200 mcgs 900 - 1000 mgs As recommended One Tablespoon	Taken with water.
7:00 pm		5% Lugol's Iodine Lemon or Lime Juice and Baking Soda Vitamin C Powder	4 drops One whole lemon/lime 1/4 to 1/2 tspn 1000 mgs	Taken all together mixed with water.
9:00 pm		Sodium Bicarbonate Lugol's Iodine	1/4 to 1/2 tspn 4 drops	Taken all together mixed with water.

The example daily schedules shown opposite are presented as a helpful guide to give people the confidence to make up daily protocol schedules according to their own needs.

Daily Protocol Schedule Notes

• Approximate conversions for powders: 1/8 tspn = 500 mgs; 1/4 tspn = 1000 mgs; 1/2 tsp = 2000 mgs.

• Borax water – 1/8 teaspoon of sodium tetraborate or borax dissolved in a litre of water, should be drunk throughout the day **as part of the above daily protocol.** Ensure that you take this borax protocol for 5 days only and then take two days off on a continual weekly basis.

• If the healing process is slow with this protocol then it is possible that more mature and hardened biofilms have formed in your body, and so you will need to use a stronger anti-biofilm protocol—either The Turpentine Protocol or The Protease Enzyme Protocol as described in Chapter 2.

• The full anti-candida diet MUST BE STRICTLY FOLLOWED with these protocols. NO SUGAR OR CARBOHYDRATES at all in the diet. Use The Health Defence Diet.

• Initially, the zinc dosage should be taken every day as stipulated in the above schedule. After two weeks this dosage should be changed to taking the zinc only once a week.

• The main nutrients that act to kill the candida and other involved pathogens throughout the body are Lugol's Iodine, borax, molybdenum, turpentine, and the alkalizing protocols.

• When starting the Lugol's Iodine protocol, you should initially start with smaller dosages and work up to the proper dose. Start small and go slow. Some people I've helped took over 30 drops of LI per day without any problems at all—this higher dosage helped them to heal their own candida problems remarkably quickly.

• Both supplementing the candida-kill remedies and supplementing the detox remedies might well create a die-off (Herxheimer) reaction or detox healing crisis. If this is the case then you can either reduce the dosages of both the candida-kill and detox remedies appropriately or you can pulse the dose—take the full dosages recommended just once every 3 days until your healing crisis improves. Read about detox and die-off or Herx reactions at the beginning of this chapter.

• Apple cider vinegar can be substituted for the lemon/lime alkalizing remedy if preferred.

• Niacin triggers the "niacin flush", which might be uncomfortable for some. Taking an aspirin 30 mins before taking niacin will reduce the flush. If the effects of the niacin flush are unbearable then just take the niacinamide (no flush) form instead. Niacin, in my opinion, is much better because it opens up the blood vessels (causing the flush), thus helping to more actively distribute the protocol nutrients to all areas of the body.

• Molybdenum – Ted recommends 10 mgs to 25 mgs of sodium molybdate a day taken for two weeks only. But buying sodium molybdate in these higher dosage amounts can be difficult. So it is perhaps best to use the 900 mcg dosage (the maximum allowed RDA allowed) three times a day as advised above.

• Vitamin C should be taken as sodium ascorbate. Calcium ascorbate should be avoided.

• The best forms of supplements to take are pure powders because they have no additives, caking-agents or calcium. The worst supplements to take are the hard tablets. This is the reason why I do not favour multivitamin tablets. *All should be supplemented at their advised dosages (not RDA dosages) within the protocols.* Smaller RDA dosages (in multivitamins) are simply ineffective.

• If you suspect parasite involvement with your candida problem, then take Hulda Clark's Parasite Cleanse for a month. This involves supplementing wormwood, black walnut extract and clove powder. This remedy, with ingredients, is easily found on the internet.

• If you also have stomach/gastric problems such as GERD, gastritis, esophagitis etc. then I would strongly recommend that you additionally supplement protease enzymes with betaine HCL at mealtimes to help resolve these issues.

Protocol Adjustments

It may become necessary to adjust your protocols – particularly the candida-kill remedies and the detox remedies – due to the Herxheimer or detox effects and reactions when you initially begin this protocol. If at the start of this protocol you suffer a severe healing crisis, then you must either reduce the dosages of the candida-kill or detox remedies to your own bearable preference or you can simply pulse the full dose of these nutrients once every three days.

Since each sufferer's health condition is different and each of us will be at different stages of candida infection as well as having different amounts of poisons and heavy metals in their bodies because of differing diets, common sense would simply dictate that these adjustments to the protocols may frequently be necessary. We are not clones and there is no one-size-fits-all with respect to dosages and frequency, so you alone must decide how to handle these problems. As a helpful aid, and if you still have questions to ask about this protocol, then I would advise that you ask your question on the Latest Post blog of EarthClinic.com where you will be able to obtain further answers to your questions about this protocol.

CHAPTER 4

The Anti-Candida Diet

The following diet is a nutritional guide and is not really a diet at all. A diet suggests that, one day, you will come off the diet. Therefore this diet is really a Way of Eating for Life. So it really should be more specifically regarded as a defensive way of eating that both helps to protect and alkalize your body. This diet advice can also be easily incorporated into other ordinary Western diets or even with organic, alkaline or vegetarian diets—where the same guidelines will apply. This diet is also recommended for problems like cancer, acid body, candida etc. on Earth Clinic. We offer it here because it is a very useful and necessary complement to the anti-candida protocols, since this way of eating helps to alkalize, detox and to protect your body from the effects of chemically processed foods.

All the same, this diet is only meant as a set of guidelines to educate. It is therefore up to the reader or candida sufferer how he or she interprets and applies it. However, if you are ill with a particularly serious illness like systemic candida, then the full diet will be necessary and must be fully and strictly applied.

The main dangers of the modern processed food diet may be adequately described by comparing this diet with our more natural, older diets. The older diets – pre-1850 – were more natural in all respects, with healthier unpolluted soils and no added chemicals or chemical processing involvement. As a result of this older food diet there were, statistically, far less persistent occurrences of chronic, autoimmune or idiopathic diseases like heart disease, cancer, diabetes, arteriosclerosis, osteoporosis, obesity, Alzheimer's, Parkinson's Disease, Chronic Fatigue Syndrome, fibromyalgia, depression etc. The keyword here is "natural". See the diagram below.

Old Food Cycle (pre 1850)

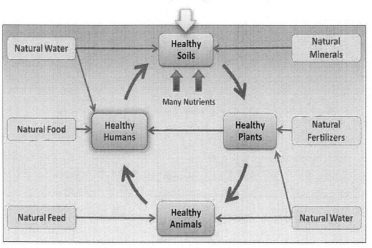

Thus when compared to the Old Food Cycle, the Modern Food Cycle could hardly, even in the kindest possible terms, be described as a natural, healthy diet. See the diagram below:

Modern Food Cycle

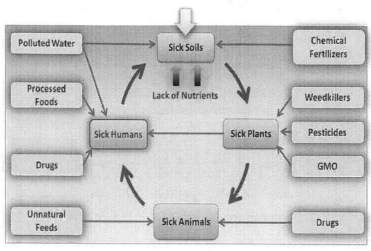

The Health Defence Diet

1. NO SUGAR. Candida, viruses and all pathogens feed off sugar, which promotes their rapid growth and spread. When too much sugar is eaten constantly every day, this habit also works to greatly lower the immune system's capability to fight disease. In particular, diseases such as cancer grow rapidly in the presence of the fructose found in fruits, and to survive they need glucose.

2. Reduce carbohydrate intake. The Western diet is effectively an energy dense but nutrient deficient diet in terms of minerals and vitamins. Therefore for sugar-loving diseases like candida, carbohydrates are banned because they so easily convert to sugar in the body. If you can, eat carbohydrates that have a low glycemic index, which are digested and absorbed slowly in the body and which do not cause high sugar spikes in the body. These sugar spikes tend to bring down the immune system and feed the invading pathogens as well. Also beware that the Glycemic Index doesn't measure the type of sugar so is not a perfect measure or guide to go by.

2. No junk food allowed. Junk food contains way too much refined salt, MSG, vegetable oils and other additives. All bad.

3. No vegetable oils in the diet. Vegetable oils oxidize fairly quickly on the shelf from sunlight and very rapidly at high heat because they are polyunsaturated (weak chemical bonds) fats. Most vegetable oils nowadays are also made from an unnatural chemical process. As far back as 1962, Dr Denham Harman, a Nobel Prize winner who discovered the anti-oxidant nature of vitamins, proved in his famous experiments in feeding mice vegetable oils with their food, that chemically processed vegetable oils or polyunsaturated oils significantly contribute to causing cancer. So, better to use a saturated fat like virgin coconut oil (VCO) or even grass-fed lard for cooking. Saturated fats are more stable oils that do not oxidize easily and are also good for you.

Many vegetarian websites quote *The Okinawan Diet* as their reason for a vegetables-only eating regimen being best for you, which is inaccurate.

If you read the book, *The Okinawan Diet* – which carefully defines this diet through the writers' research – the Okinawans generally used pork offal and pork fat in all their healthy cooking; and, in their pre-WW2 diet they never used whole grain bread, olive oil, soy milk, apples, or yogurt.

When I had systemic candida and started taking coconut oil, my terrible daily constipation and bloating issues completely disappeared in about two weeks and my toilet habits became regular again. VCO is very healthy for your body and intestines. I only ever cook with VCO now, and it has actually helped me to lose weight.

Since the 1960s, baby-foods have been using only coconut oil for their cooked products, and those in the hospital with intestinal trauma are usually fed with food cooked in coconut oil as well. This is because VCO helps to protect the intestines and the body while also being anti-bacterial, anti-viral and anti-fungal.

4. No soda pop. Apart from containing sugar, high fructose corn syrup (HFCS), fructose and aspartame, sweet soda drinks also contain carbonic and phosphoric acids as well as halogens like fluorides in their mix—all of which only work to acidify your body. Furthermore, HFCS often contains mercury and poisonous chemicals like glutaraldehyde, which is normally used as a poisonous industrial cleaner.

5. No artificial sweeteners–no aspartame, sucralose or saccharine. Aspartame is acidifying. It is also an excitotoxin that helps to destroy your central nervous system. In our bodies, aspartame metabolizes into formaldehyde and methanol, which is also a poison. (In the old days people used stills to make their own illicit distilled alcoholic beverages and if they were not careful in their process methanol would form. This wood alcohol or methanol is very poisonous and as little as 10 ml would be enough to cause permanent blindness.) Sucralose is a chlorinated hydrocarbon that, in tests, causes a shrunken thymus, enlarged kidneys, abortion and low fetal weights, as these areas are all sensitive to chlorine compounds in hydrocarbon forms. Saccharine, even a moderate dose, can increase the incidence of tumors in people with cancer.

6. Eat chicken, fish and meats in small amounts. Proteins – meats – eaten in excessive quantities are acidifying as we get older, since our bodies have difficulty digesting them. Proteins should preferably be partially cooked to ease the breaking down of proteins.

7. No baked goods like bread, cakes, pastries, etc. In the '70s the FDA, in their wisdom, allowed the use of bromide and bromates in bread-making instead of iodine. Bromine weakens the immune system and encourages an acid body state. Wheat also contains gluten and alloxan, the latter a poison that can help to destroy the pancreas and causes diabetes over time.

8. Add coriander/cilantro and green tea to your diet routine. In your diet, include a handful of raw, chopped coriander leaf (also called cilantro) in a salad three times a week and drink green tea 2-3 times a day. Maintaining this regimen for a month will successfully remove most heavy metals from your body.

9. No canned products in the diet. Bisphenol A (BPA) is a component in the plastic that lines canned goods, and is very bad for you. It acts as a pseudo-estrogen – a female hormone – and upsets hormone balance, thereby weakening the immune system.

10. No calcium, which means no dairy products. No milk, no cheese, no yoghurt, no ice cream etc. Avoid all calcium fortified foods. Excess calcium encourages acidity throughout the body and particularly in the tissue cells where it tends to calcify mitochondria causing loss of energy and myalgia. In 1970, the recommended calcium to magnesium ratio was 4:1. Then it became 2:1 in the 1990s. I'm guessing that, probably in another 10 years, these same RDA experts will recommend a calcium to magnesium ratio of 1:1. I recommend taking no calcium supplementation in your diet because Western foods are all over-fortified with calcium now. Calcium causes acidity inside the cells when taken in excess and when magnesium is lacking in the diet. Magnesium regulates calcium in the body.

11. No fruits. In general most fruits contain citric acid and sugar—especially the citrus fruits. In a healthy body that can cope with the acid and sugars from fruits it is fine to eat fruits in moderation. But if you are ill with an acid-loving and sugar-loving disease like cancer, then any acidic or sugary food like fruits will actually promote its spread because eating fruits uses up your alkaline body bicarbonates during digestion. This further weakens the immune system, increases acidity and glucose levels in the blood and helps diseases like candida to dominate the body. You can use fruit extracts that don't contain fructose, such as red wine extract, grapeseed extract etc.

12. No Monosodium Glutamate (MSG). MSG is disallowed for the same reasons as aspartame. The antidote to MSG is taurine amino acid, which is mainly found in fish.

13. Avoid GMO foods. The most common GMO food is actually wheat. But there is also soy, beet and corn GMO. All soy products made from a chemical process – including soy sauce, tofu etc. – should be avoided. But any soy products made from a natural and organic fermentation process are allowed. If you buy soya products like soya milk, make sure it is organic and contains soya flour. If it contains soya protein then it has been made from a chemical process and also might be GMO (especially in the US).

14. Avoid distilled water and tap water. Distilled water is "dead water"—it completely lacks the important minerals that natural spring-water contains. If you drink distilled water, this will actually act to pull important minerals out of your body during digestion. Tap water nowadays – due to water shortages – is recycled and chemically processed from sewage (especially in cities) and stored in reservoirs that are fed from water tables polluted with agricultural fertilizers and pesticides, so goodness knows what evil goodies tap water contains. Enough said I think. Drink fresh mineral or spring water or create your own mineral water instead. You should always drink 1-2 glasses of water at mealtimes. This helps digestion and will improve your urine conductivity reading, provided your body minerals are in balance.

15. Use sea salt rather than refined table salt. Use sea salt for all your cooking and eating needs. Sea salt contains many other beneficial natural minerals, is alkaline, and also aids nutrient absorption and acts like a protective antibiotic in the body, which helps to protect the intestines and liver. Sea salt is also far more alkaline than refined table salt, which is normally acidic.

16. Try to avoid all (chemically) processed food. Try to eat foods that are made from natural processes without excess heating or use of chemicals. Read food labels carefully before you buy.

17. Eat your big meals early. Whenever you eat your meals, it is always best to eat bigger meals at breakfast and lunch. Your evening dinner should be eaten early at about 5:00 pm because shortly after this time, your body goes into another mode. This mode slows down digestion, making it inefficient, which actually impairs digestion, such that large amounts of food can end up sitting and stagnating in your intestines for up to 12 hours. This results in acidity build-up, pathogen growth and poisons being absorbed into the body from the intestines. Better as a habit to eat a much smaller quantity of food at dinner to ensure healthy and complete digestion of food before sleep.

18. Enjoy your meals! When you eat food, don't always rush and over-stuff yourself, as this can lead to poor, inefficient digestion and acid intestines. There is always a lag from when you feel hungry to when your hunger is satisfied, but if you eat too fast you will eat more than your body needs, and this is not good for you. Eat your food slower, chew food thoroughly, and drink plenty of water at mealtimes for proper digestion. The Chinese – and Okinawans – normally eat until they feel 70% full, then they stop. This is a good, simple dietary practice.

CHAPTER 5

Preventative Aftercare

Since, as I have already described, candida infections and persistence are greatly assisted by a poor diet, then after you have successfully resolved your own candida problems, it makes sense to change your diet from a processed food diet to a healthier diet that is more nutrient dense rather than energy dense. To this end, you should adhere to the *Health Defence Diet* given in this book. And the degree or strictness to which you follow this diet, I leave up to you. But just remember that a continuous adherence to a poor diet will, over time, undoubtedly help to promote not only candida but other serious chronic diseases as well.

To be honest, my own more realistic philosophy on health and protecting the body is that eating poor quality processed food is simply unavoidable nowadays. I like to go to gatherings and parties and go out to restaurants to enjoy the company of friends. Who doesn't? Sometimes people have to travel in their jobs and eat fast food because there is nothing else available. So it is quite difficult to avoid processed food these days. That is why my own day to day health regimen is necessarily ongoing and defensive. In fact it is a habit with me now.

Another useful strategy is to have a hair analysis. Having a hair analysis done will tell you exactly what minerals and vitamins are lacking in your diet and will also tell you what heavy metals and other poisons you have in excess in your body. This is a good start point because this allows you to more accurately fine-tune your own daily aftercare protocols to the results of your own hair analysis.

My own daily, weekly and monthly protocols protect against the following:

Lack of Minerals and Vitamins in the Diet – Humic acid (minerals and trace minerals), sea salt (minerals and trace minerals), B vitamins, vitamin C (gram dosages), desiccated liver tablets (the best all-around source of minerals, vitamins and amino acids – and cheap!), ALA, Lugol's Iodine, selenium, zinc, magnesium.

Heavy Metals and Other Poisons in the Diet – Humic acid (twice weekly), chlorella (daily), turpentine (weekly or monthly), sodium thiosulfate (weekly), Lugol's Iodine (daily), alkalizing (daily).

Anti-Candida, Anti-Pathogen (strengthens the immune system) – Turpentine, borax, Lugol's Iodine (daily), humic acid (bi-weekly), magnesium chloride (daily), alkalizing (daily), sea salt.

Liver and Kidney Health – ALA, selenium and milk thistle on a daily basis.

Eating a Healthy Non-Processed Food Diet. This is common sense.

As you can see, the above aftercare regimen is not such a huge protocolwhich just addresses my own particular needs. You will also notice that many of the above nutrients address more than one problem, which is also quite useful. The aftercare protocol also deliberately contains a large amount of critical anti-oxidants for the body that are very necessary in our already nutrient-depleted diets.

My own continuous day-to-day candida aftercare strategy is simply based on thoroughly protecting the intestines, liver, kidneys and thyroid gland. If you adopt this strategy then:

- Nutritional pathways into the body will be healthy and assured.
- General metabolism becomes more efficient.
- Body alkalinity is increased and maintained at healthy levels.
- The body's hormones are more properly regulated and balanced.
- Mood is improved, depression reduced.
- The blood is purified and so the proper transport of nutrients will also be assured.
- Energy levels will be greatly improved.
- Fat build-up and poisons in the blood are reduced with the liver protected and assisted.

- The excretory pathways are also assured and healthy.
- The body's immune system is greatly strengthened.

Since adopting the above candida aftercare strategy and for the last six or seven years I have not been ill with any infectious disease (even with flu epidemics in my area), my heart and energy are both good and I have no aches and pains. I have no auto-immune or chronic problems. I'm 63 years old and feel much younger than my years. But when I had systemic candida, as I've already mentioned, my health was a very different story indeed.

CHAPTER 6

General Discussion on Health

"As the philosopher Schopenhauer said, 'All truth goes through three stages. First, it is ridiculed. Then, it is violently opposed. Finally, it is accepted as self-evident.' Within five years, people who ignore the importance of yeast-related illness will be in the same camp with those in the Flat-Earth Society."
—Dr William Shaw

In finally reaching closure with the subject of candida, I suppose the obvious question to ask about this book is, "There are so many anti-candida protocols being sold out there, what makes your protocols more special, useful or successful than all the other anti-candida protocols?" A fair question which I have indeed thought about and spent some time considering. First of all, to be clear, I'm not selling anything except the ideas in this book and I very much doubt whether I will achieve millionaire status through its sales. Secondly, I sell no pills, herbs or extracts at exorbitant prices for self-profit and I have no personal website dedicated to my own self-promotion or self-aggrandizement.

My real and ultimate purpose for writing this book was to simply reveal, as much and as honestly as possible, all the most competent, research-driven and alternative strategies and methods that have been successfully proven to cure candida problems. I also had long-term systemic candida and managed to successfully and completely cure it myself by using *The Main Anti-Candida Protocol* given in this book. I have also read hundreds of testimonials from people who have either successfully or unsuccessfully treated their own candida problems, so I think that I have had a particularly good grounding and view as to what works and what really doesn't work against candida. This is why the information contained in this book is so important. Because these protocols work. Much of the information in this book is also unique, untold or unrealized and, if nothing else, the facts herein should fully arm candida sufferers with more than sufficient knowledge and proper facts to help them to fully understand how they can ultimately defeat their own difficult fungal disease.

So how do the remedies and protocols in this book stack up against other anti-candida protocols that are out there?

Speaking generally, many other candida protocols use undecylenic acid, a derivative of castor oil, as one of the main candida attack remedies. Undecylenic acid is a highly useful anti-pathogen. But from the research, although undecylenic acid has certainly been found to inhibit the morphing of candida from the yeast form to the more virulent fungal or mycelial form, inhibiting candida really does not fulfill my own criteria for achieving a proper cure. Unfortunately, inhibiting candida does not mean kill ALL the candida. And what if you already have the systemic fungal form, which is perhaps still breeding happily away and spreading in the blood, tissues and organs **outside the intestines**? Will undecylenic acid kill and eradicate the body-wide fungal candida form as well? Will undecylenic acid have candida-killing efficacy in both the intestines as well as throughout ALL regions of the body? There are too many unanswered questions using undecylenic acid as the main candida-killing ingredient in an anti-candida regimen.

Nystatin is another anti-fungal that is regularly used by the medical profession and healers against fungal problems like candida. Supplementing nystatin can be quite useful but will only ever eradicate candida locally, having little efficacy against the more widely dispersed fungal or disseminated form of candida. This is because nystatin is known to be very poorly absorbed into the blood from the intestines.[136,137] Nystatin also has a high toxicity profile, which is why there are no injectable or IV forms. So if you have the systemic fungal form of candida already so widely dispersed throughout your body (outside the intestines) then nystatin will simply not work because the untouched disseminated fungal form will just repopulate the intestines after a while and the candida infection will keep returning until the candida is eventually able to fully adjust to nystatin—and then nystatin becomes a useless protocol. Many people also use Diflucan (fluconazole) against various forms of candida. I initially used Diflucan three times against my own candida and it had no effect whatsoever—it didn't even help my constipation. And, from all the health blogs that I've read concerning candida and the use of Diflucan, if you do actually manage to get rid of the candida from your intestines using Diflucan, it is normally the case – as with using nystatin – that candida comes roaring back with a vengeance a month or so later.

Chitinase is another highly touted component of many anti-candida protocols and is a chitin-digesting enzyme that is supposed to attack and dissolve the candida cell walls (made of chitin). Unfortunately and from all the research that I've so far read, candida is apparently easily able to adjust to or hide from chitinase, rendering it useless as a cure. Candida can easily hide inside biofilms that are made of fibrin—not made of cellulose or chitin. So these are the main reasons why supplementing chitinase for candida problems is not always successful. Chitinase will simply not work consistently well unless you get rid of the candida biofilms first.

I have also studied many of the candida cure regimens by candida experts on the internet and have found the majority of these protocols to be completely lacking effectiveness in ridding candida from the body for good (with no return of candida). The main reasons why these other anti-candida regimens fail is because of a wide lack of understanding on how candida behaves as an organism. In most of these other protocols there is no overt emphasis or recognition that candida is a dimorphic organism – both a fungus and a yeast – and there seems to be no appreciation at all how candida uses biofilms to so successfully hide and protect itself from anti-fungals and anti-microbials. The majority of these protocols contain no sufficiently effective anti-biofilm ingredients and so the candida is able to hide safely in these biofilms, and that's another reason why the candida keeps returning time and time again. These other protocols also do not usually contain molybdenum within their protocols, which has been fully proven through research to both kill candida and neutralize and safely remove the dangerous candida mycotoxins in the blood.

In these other protocols, there appears to be no acceptance nor any understanding on how candida is always associated with other bacterial co-infections or diseases. These are never addressed in other protocols – all their protocols ever do is try to kill the candida – with no attempt to eradicate other pathogens. And there is absolutely no appreciation about how effective iodine and borax are against pathogens (including candida) and little, if any, understanding on how helpful alkalizing is against candida despite all the research evidence that is out there.

In my own efforts to try to help people with serious candida issues, I have also come to realize that, from a human decision point of view, certain other problems can arise that will hamper a cure. I have found several human reasons why people fail with their anti-candida protocols due to their own incorrect approach or attitude, and these reasons for failure are defined here.

Lack of proper knowledge concerning the behaviour of candida
Choice of protocols or nutrients based solely on convenience factors
Lack of determination or willpower to follow the protocols correctly
Not strictly following the anti-candida diet

In this book, I have tried to thoroughly explain and describe clearly the reasons for using all the nutrients within the protocols in order to help people finally resolve their candida problems, but time and time again, some sufferers opt not to use the whole multi-protocol as advised. Instead these sufferers prefer to cherry-pick only one or two of the remedies in the protocol in the greatly mistaken belief that they will be cured. I have also found that any candida protocol will almost certainly fail, from a human point of view, mainly due to lack of understanding or lack of determination or for convenience factors or for reasons of sheer indulgence (continual adherence to bad dietary and lifestyle habits). As in life, if you do not have the willpower, determination and focus to fight your own candida problems, then no-one will be able to help you and you will most likely fail to achieve your goal. So if you want to successfully resolve your own serious candida problems, then you should use all the anti-candida strategies and nutrients contained within the protocols consistently, on a daily basis and as advised. In other words, there are no shortcuts.

In this book, I've also made it quite clear that my own favourite candida-kill combination is iodine, borax (sodium tetraborate) and alkalizing. For me, this combination has been very successful at killing all the candida throughout the body and getting rid of it for good. What makes Lugol's Iodine so good at killing candida and other pathogen species? Quite simply, there is no other single chemical element or substance on this planet that kills such a wide range of pathogens (including yeast/fungus) with the same speed as iodine. Because of this speed-of-kill factor no pathogen can ever adjust to iodine because they just don't have the time to do so. Iodine prevents viruses, bacteria and fungi from attaching to cells in order to feed and to breed. Iodine immediately and quickly dissolves the tyrosine and histidine amino acid layers, which are always exposed and present in the folds of most pathogen cell walls. Iodine does not attack human cells because the tyrosine and histidine layers in human cells are safely hidden away. Iodine is an anti-pathogen and anti-fungal that acts throughout the body to kill candida—in all regions of the body and not just in the intestines. Iodine also acts as a surfactant capable of disrupting and dispelling biofilms to more completely expose the candida and associated pathogens. Iodine is furthermore a very efficient detoxer of heavy metals, halides and other poisons in the body.

Nevertheless, borax is perhaps the ultimate fungal killer for similar reasons to iodine. Borax (sodium tetraborate) has the same body toxicity profile as common table salt. Borax also efficiently kills mycoplasma and certain other bacteria, and borax is alkaline. The alkalizing remedies act to hugely reinforce the protocol by setting up the worst possible environment for the acid-loving candida. What do people use to clean their fridges and to eradicate mold and fungus? Sodium bicarbonate!

On reflection and after defining my own experiences and self-practiced views on health, I freely admit that I am a wholehearted believer in the efficacy of self-treatment with natural and alternative methods that have been developed and have successfully persisted for thousands of years, whereas the relatively newborn allopathic approach of modern medicine and drugs, with so many merely palliative treatments, together with their somewhat arrogant insistence and propaganda that they are the only real experts on illness and disease, would seem to be consistently contradicted by their continuing inability and failure to understand, let alone fail to consistently cure, so many serious autoimmune and idiopathic diseases such as cancer, heart disease, arteriosclerosis, osteoporosis, arthritis, obesity, diabetes, Alzheimer's disease and even the common cold, just to name a few. And all this failure, despite well over one hundred years of intense modern medical research and decades of ongoing funding in the billions from governments and charities.

In my own ongoing study of research papers I also came to learn, in fair detail, modern medicine's method for developing drugs. This method never varies and seems to me to also be a sadly inadequate process. This strictly defined process begins by researching just one chemical – such as a newly discovered natural plant chemical – intensely in relation to its efficacy against one particular disease or illness; and if this plant chemical does indeed have positive healing effects on a particular disease, then the next development stage is for drugs research to invent an equivalent but patentable chemical with the same or similar healing properties as the plant chemical. This latter stage is mandatory. Notably, if they cannot invent an equivalent patentable chemical then their research is usually secretly dumped, even if the natural plant chemical they originally found does indeed have positive benefits against a particular disease. The next stage, after successfully patenting the drug, is to further test it for efficacy and safety using double blind placebo testing on animals and then medical trials with humans. This proof of efficacy and safety is undertaken, amazingly, by the very drugs company that invented the drug in the first place (what about proper independent checks, balances and transparency to avoid biased results?). And after satisfactorily passing the FDA requirements, the new drug is then released for use and open to further peer research review.

The biggest failing in the above standardized research process for inventing and proving the efficacy and safety of any new drug is that the whole proving process is so heavily constrained and dependent upon whether a patentable equivalent chemical can be found. Therefore this aspect alone must substantially limit the abilities of this type of drugs research to create more useful drugs in the future. And the expense of proving the efficacy and safety of any single drug, it must be said, is also so horrifically expensive verging on the utterly ridiculous. As an example, one kilogram of vincristine, an older cancer chemo drug that is still being used against cancer, costs about $20 million to buy today. That means that 1 gram of vincristine will cost any unfortunate cancer sufferer $20,000 (not including hospital costs and payments).

Regarding the specific use of healing herbs, alternative medicine fully recognizes and relies much more upon the beneficial synergistic chemical activity arising from the hundreds of natural chemicals usually found in a healing plant or herb and does not just rely on one single chemical component. Synergism, when used to describe the action of the beneficial chemicals in a plant as a group, means that the healing activity of the combined natural chemical components of the plant is far greater than the sum of its chemical parts. Unfortunately, the standard medical research process has no ability to use the synergism of chemicals in plants like this as a viable strategy to resolve illness and disease because of both the vast complexity and expense of first proving the synergism of all these plant chemicals and then having to find equivalent patentable chemicals in order to reclaim the research expense involved in satisfying the stringent FDA requirements for acceptance. This is why, as far as I am able to ascertain, modern medical research and the FDA acceptance process is such a very constrained road to follow in terms of any positive future prospects for continued drug viability and success.

I have also noticed from certain independent research that either directly contradicts or threatens long established drugs research or research that offends any one of their major money-making drugs industries – such as those drugs used for heart disease, cancer, Alzheimer's disease, arthritis, diabetes, osteoporosis or depression – that the worldwide medical peer review committees are so easily able to suppress the findings from the more honest and less biased independent research by deliberate exclusion from the peer review process. If there are no peer reviews for new research findings, then there will be no recognition or acceptance of any successful independent research discoveries within the research community. That's the rule. In fact this happened to Linus Pauling, who was perhaps the foremost chemist of the last century and whose work that earned the Nobel Prize in chemistry changed the very way we now think about the nature of chemical bonding. Pauling's research methods were also meticulous, unassailable in accuracy and logic and consequently highly regarded by the research community. His new findings on the positive healing effects of gram oral amounts of lysine and vitamin C on arteriosclerosis and heart disease – a remarkably simple and cheap remedy – with the more than probable prospect that certain drugs companies and medical concerns would, as a result of Pauling's research, lose significant amounts of profit revenue from the sale of statins as well as stent and bypass operations, forced these medical research review committees in the US to react in the only way they knew how. And so, with no other recourse or any accurate evidence to rely upon, they haughtily declared that Linus Pauling was not a microbiologist – he was a chemist – and that he had no business involving himself in research on heart disease as an unqualified microbiological researcher and therefore his research on heart disease was invalid and should be ignored! How's that for honest logic? Linus Pauling, in several of his books and ever the gentleman, was always gently scathing of these heavily steered and biased allopathic opinions concerning his research.

Many people these days also seem to be completely satisfied with doctors only ever accommodating their disease using palliative treatments—just treating their symptoms (as is almost always the case for most auto-immune or idiopathic diseases). Patients certainly seem happy enough for doctors to only ever treat their idiopathic (medical meaning: we haven't got one clue what causes your disease) or auto-immune (medical meaning: blame this disease entirely on the immune system) symptoms with evermore palliative drugs. Above all, this book preaches cure and resolution rather than disease or pathogen "accommodation" by just treating symptoms. There is simply no other honest way in my own opinion. Everyone should always aim and strive unceasingly for a direct cure no matter what awful disease they happen to have.

I would further like to add that no-one should ever trust or be satisfied with any drug, remedy or treatment that obviously doesn't ultimately work to actually **cure** your candida problems, *no matter who insists that such a drug or remedy should work!* Find out for yourself and use your own God-given judgment. That makes you the judge and expert – not the doctor or any so-called health expert – because you are the only person who can **feel** whether the drug or treatment is working or not. And if you are not satisfied with your doctor's approach or treatment and your own doctor is unaccommodating, then I would suggest that you read Andrew Saul's most excellent book, *Fire Your Doctor!* for some helpful advice and clarity.

In the end, I guess that you could also call me somewhat of a libertarian in my own views and treatment of illness and disease. Real understanding of disease and cure is based upon true and accurate knowledge—real honest-to-God facts from honest research. I truly believe that everyone has a right to good health and that the decisions that we must all individually make concerning proper treatments for our ills and diseases are so hugely important. That is why, in the final judgment, the ultimate responsibility regarding final outcomes from decisions concerning disease solutions must belong solely to us – our own free will and choice – and does not belong singularly within the realms of doctors and the modern medical profession. In other words, that each and every one of us must critically but gladly take full responsibility for decisions about our own lifelong health and happiness.

Finally, in closing and in conclusion, please be particularly careful and especially discerning as to who you entrust with your own serious health problems. Health is a particularly rare and precious commodity these days. Bear in mind that the final outcome and responsibility for your own good health and wellbeing belongs only to you and nobody else.

RESOURCE INDEX

Resources and References

As a helpful aid to a deeper understanding of candida as a disease and as evidence to support the efficacy of the ideas and protocols in this book, I have listed a large body of evidence, from both standard research and from alternative medicine sources, that will help the reader to generally increase his or her understanding and knowledge on candida as a pathogen.

If the reader has the need to find out more, questions may also be asked on the Latest Post blog section of the *EarthClinic.com* website.

References

Candida

1. Truss CO, *The Missing Diagnosis*; The Missing Diagnosis: 1983.

2. Crook WG, et al, *The Yeast Connection: A Medical Breakthrough*; Jackson Professional Books Inc: Tennessee, 1991.

3. Crook WG, *The Yeast Connection and Women's Health*; Professional Books Inc: Jackson, Tennessee, 2003.

4. Grisanti RJ, Understanding the Candida Infection. Your Medical Detective online, 2013. http://www.yourmedicaldetective.com/public/254.cfm

5. Calderone RA, et al, Virulence factors of Candida Albicans. *Trends Microbiol.*; 9 (7): 327-35; July 2001. http://www.ncbi.nlm.nih.gov/pubmed/11435107

6. Walter Last, *Overcoming Candida: A Guide to Self Healing*; Austpac Productions: Moss Vale, Australia, Revised Edition, 2012.

7. Moore CW, The Candida Syndrome: Health Nemesis or Myth? Natural Life Magazine online. *http://www.naturallifemagazine.com/9804/candida.htm*

8. Truss CO, Metabolic Abnormalities in Patients with Chronic Candidiasis: The Acetaldehyde Hypothesis. *Jour of Orthomol Psych;* 13 (2); 1984. *http://www.orthomolecular.org/library/jom/1984/pdf/1984-v13n02-p066.pdf*

9. Weiss J, The Candida Aldehyde Detox Pathway And The Molybdenum Connection. Candidapage online, Oct 2009. *http://candidapage.com/aldehyde.shtml*

10. Truss OC, Tissue Injury Induced by Candida Albicans: Mental and Neurologic Manifestations. *Orthomol. Psychiatry,* 7 (1); pp 17-37; 1978. *http://orthomolecular.org/library/jom/1978/pdf/1978-v07n01-p017.pdf*

11. Trowbridge JP, Walker M, *The Yeast Syndrome: How to Help Your Doctor Identify & Treat the Real Cause of Your Yeast-Related Illness*; Bantam Books, New York, 1986.

12. Bakker E, Why Do Doctors Often Miss Candida Diagnosis? YeastInfection. org online, July 13, 2013. *http://www.yeastinfection.org/why-do-practitioners-often-miss-the-candida-diagnosis/*

13. Evans SE, Coping with Candida Infections. *Proc Am Thorac Soc;* 7 (3); pp 197-203; May 2010. *http://pats.atsjournals.org/content/7/3/197.full.pdf*

14. Ray TL, Systemic Candidiasis, *Dermatol Clin;* 7(2): pp 259-68; April 1989. *http://www.ncbi.nlm.nih.gov/pubmed/2670371*

15. Jehn U, Managing fungal and viral infection in the immunocompromised host, Recent Results. *Cancer Res;* 108: pp 61-70; 1988. *http://www.ncbi.nlm.nih.gov/pubmed/3051213*

16. Anane S, et al, Biological diagnosis of systemic candidiasis: difficulties and future prospects. *Pathol Biol (Paris)*; 55 (5): pp 262-72; June 2007. *http://www.ncbi.nlm.nih.gov/pubmed/16698196*

17. Gaby AR, Recurrent Candidiasis: One Step Forward, Still Backward. Townsend Letter for Doctors and Patients, Townsend Letter online, No 2004 v. *http://www.townsendletter.com/Nov2004/gabyeditorial1104.htm*

18. Pfaller MA, et al, Epidemiology of Invasive Candidiasis: A Persistent Public Health Problem. Dept of Epidemiology, University of Iowa, *Clin. Microbiol. Rev;* 20 (1); pp 133-163. Jan 2007. *http://cmr.asm.org/content/20/1/133.abstract*

19. DiNubile MJ, et al. Invasive candidiasis in cancer patients: Observations from a randomized clinical trial. *J. Infect;* 50 (5); pp 443-9; Jun 2005. *http://www.ncbi.nlm.nih.gov/pubmed/15907554*

20. Hopfer RL, et al. Radiometric detection of yeasts in blood cultures of cancer patients. *Journ. of Clin. Micro;* pp 329-331; Sept 1980. *http://jcm.asm.org/content/12/3/329.full.pdf*

21. Degregorio MW, et al, Candida infections in patients with acute leukemia: Ineffectiveness of nystatin prophylaxis and relationship between oropharyngeal and systemic candidiasis. Science Direct online; *Cancer.* 50 (12): pp 2780–2784, Dec 1982. *http://onlinelibrary.wiley.com/doi/10.1002/1097-0142 1982121550:12%3C2780::AID-CNCR2820501215%3E3.0.CO;2-P/abstract*

22. Novey HS, et al, Prevalence of Aspergillus and Candida Precipitins in Renal Dialysis and Transplant Patients. Informa Care online, *Renal Fail;* Vol. 3, No. 4, Pages 349-360; 1979. *http://informahealthcare.com/doi/abs/10.3109/0886022790 9063952?journalCode=rnf*

23. Lipsitch M, et al, Antimicrobial Use and Antimicrobial Resistance: A Population Perspective. CDC, *Emerg. Infect.* Dis; 84; p. 347-354; April 2002. *http://www.ncbi.nlm.nih.gov/pmc/articles*

24. Kumamoto AC, Candida biofilms. *Dept Mol. Biol,* Tufts Uni., Boston: 5 (6); pp 608-611; Dec 2002. *http://www.sciencedirect.com/science/article/pii/S1369527402003715*

25. Leroy LO, et al, Epidemiology, management, and risk factors for death of invasive Candida infections in critical care: A multicenter, prospective, observational study in France. Critical Care Medicine online, *CCM;* Vol 37; Issue 5; pp 1612-1618; May 2009. *http://journals.lww.com/ccmjournal/Abstract/2009/05000/Epidemiology,_management,_and_risk_factors_for.10.aspx*

26. Krčméry V, et al, Documented Fungal Infections after Prophylaxis or Therapy with Wide Spectrum Antibiotics: Relationship Between Certain Fungal Pathogens and Particular Antimicrobials. *Journal of Chemotherapy* (Florence, Italy); 115: pp 385-390; 1999. *http://europepmc.org/abstract/MED/10632385*

27. Picazo JJ, et al, Candidemia in the critically ill patient. Int J *Antimicrob Agents;* 32 Suppl 2: pp 83-5; Nov 2008. *http://www.ncbi.nlm.nih.gov/pubmed/19013345*

28. Delisle MS, et al, The Clinical Significance of Candida Colonization of Respiratory Tract Secretions in Critically Ill Patients. *Can Respir Jour;* 183; May-June 2011. *http://www.ncbi.nlm.nih.gov/pmc/articles/PMC3328877/*

29. Dorko E, et al, Fungal diseases of the respiratory tract. *Folia Microbiologica Jour;* Volume 47, Issue 3, pp 302-304; June 2002. *http://www.springerlink.com/content/a59677t885011304/*

30. Knutsen AP, et al, Fungi and allergic lower respiratory tract diseases. *Jour of Allergy and Clinical Immunology;* Volume 129, Issue 2, pp 280-291, Feb 2012. http://www.jacionline.org/article/S0091-6749 1102939-3/abstract

31. Santelmann H, et al, Yeast metabolic products, yeast antigens and yeasts as possible triggers for irritable bowel syndrome. *Euro Journal of Gastro & Hepatol.* Dis; 171: pp 21-6; Jan 2005. *http://www.ncbi.nlm.nih.gov/pubmed/15647635*

32. Cater, RE, Chronic candidiasis as a possible etiological factor in the chronic fatigue syndrome. *Medical Hypotheses;* 446: pp 507-15; June 1995. *http://www.ncbi.nlm.nih.gov/pubmed/7476598*

33. Hazen KC, Chronic Urinary Tract Infection Due to Candida *utilis. Jour Clinical Microbiol;* 373; pp 824 -827; March 1999. *http://www.ncbi.nlm.nih.gov/pmc/articles/PMC84571/*

34. Seelig MS, Mechanisms by which antibiotics increase the incidence and severity of candidiasis and alter the immunological defenses. *Bacteriol Rev;* 302: pp 442-459; June 1966. *http://www.ncbi.nlm.nih.gov/pmc/articles/PMC441005/*

35. Sendid B, et al, Anti-glycan antibodies establish an unexpected link between C.

albicans and Crohn disease. *Med Sci (Paris)*; 255: pp 473-81; 2009 May. *http://www.ncbi.nlm.nih.gov/pubmed/19480828*

36. Garst J, Yeast organisms and Prostatitis. Prostatitis Foundation online, 2002. *http://www.prostatitis.org/yeastessay.html*

Candida and Dimorphism

37. Kerridge D, Fungal Dimorphism: A Sideways Look. *Dimorphic Fungi in Biology and Medicine*; pp 3-10; 1993. *http://link.springer.com/chapter/10.1007/978-1-4615-2834-0_1*

38. Hartmann J, Pleomorphism as a Therapeutic Principle for Candida Mycoses. *SANUM-Post magazine*; 18/1992. *http://www.semmelweis.de/pdf/pdf.php?name=18_hartmann_albicansan_gbr&ext=pdf*

39. Molero G, et al, Candida albicans: genetics, dimorphism and pathogenicity. *International Microbiol*; 1: pp 95-106; 1998. *http://www.im.microbios.org/02june98/04%20Molero.pdf*

40. Mitchell AP, Dimorphism and virulence in Candida albicans. *Curr Opin Microbiol*; 16:687-92; Dec 1998. *http://www.ncbi.nlm.nih.gov/pubmed/10066539*

41. Olmtead SF, et al, Life on the edge: the clinical implications of gastrointestinal biofilm. Townsend Letter online; Oct 2009. *http://www.thefreelibrary.com/Life+on+the+edge:+the+clinical+implications+of+gas%20trointestinal+ .-a0211561662*

42. Chandra J, et al, Biofilm Formation by the Fungal Pathogen Candida albicans: Development, Architecture, and Drug Resistance. *J Bacteriol.*; 18318: pp 5385-94; Sep 2001. *http://www.ncbi.nlm.nih.gov/pubmed/11514524*

43. Ramage G, et al, Fungal biofilm resistance. *Int J Microbiol*; 528521; Feb 2012. *http://www.ncbi.nlm.nih.gov/pubmed/22518145*

44. Ramage G, et al, Candida Biofilms: an Update. *Eukarotic Cell*; 44; pp 633-638; April 2005. *http://ec.asm.org/content/4/4/633.full*

45. Douglas L J, Candida biofilms and their role in infection. *Trends Microbiol*; 111: pp 30-6; Jan 2003. *http://www.sciencedirect.com/science/article/pii/S0966842X02000021Glasgow*

46. Didilescu A, Biofilms. *Pneumologia*; 531: pp 26-30; Jan-Mar 2004. *http://www.ncbi.nlm.nih.gov/pubmed/18210718*

47. Hawser SP, et al, Resistance of Candida albicans biofilms to antifungal agents in vitro. *Antimicrob. Agents Chemotherapy*; Vol. 39 no. 9; pp 2128-2131; Sep 1995. *http://aac.asm.org/content/39/9/2128.short*

48. Baillie GS et al, Role of dimorphism in the development of Candida albicans biofilms. *Journal of Medical Microbiology online. JMM*; vol. 48 no. 7; pp 671-679; July 1999. *http://jmm.sgmjournals.org/content/48/7/671.short*

49. Sardi JC, et al, Candida species: current epidemiology, pathogenicity, biofilm formation, natural antifungal products and new therapeutic options, *J Med Microbiol.* 62 Pt 1: pp 10-24. Jan 2013. *http://www.ncbi.nlm.nih.gov/pubmed/23180477*

50. Hogan DA, Talking to Themselves: Autoregulation and Quorum Sensing in Fungi. *Eukaryot Cell*; 54: pp 613-9; Apr 2006. *http://www.ncbi.nlm.nih.gov/pubmed/16607008*

51. Nguyen D, et al, Active Starvation Responses Mediate Antibiotic Tolerance in Biofilms and Nutrient-Limited Bacteria. *Science*: Vol; 334; no. 6058; pp 982-986; Nov 2011. *http://www.sciencemag.org/content/334/6058/982*

52. Ash C, Arrest and Tolerate. *Sci. Signal.*; Vol. 4, Issue 200, pp. 328; Nov 2011. *http://stke.sciencemag.org/cgi/content/abstract/4/200/ec328*

Mixed Species Biofilms

53. Adam B, et al, Mixed species biofilms of Candida albicans and Staphylococcus epidermidis. *J Med Microbiol*; 51(4); pp 344-349; April 2002. *http://jmm.sgmjournals.org/content/51/4/344.short*

54. Thein ZM, et al, Community lifestyle of Candida in mixed biofilms: a mini review. *Mycoses*; 52 (6); pp 467-475, Nov 2009. *http://onlinelibrary.wiley.com/doi/10.1111/j.1439-0507.2009.01719.x/abstract*

The Herxheimer or Die-Off Effect

55. Pybus PK, et al, The Herxheimer Effect. The Arthritis Trust online. *http://www.arthritistrust.org/Articles/2-Case%20Histories.pdf*

Antibiotic Resistance

56. Swain F, Antibiotic resistance: Bacteria are winning the war. UK Guardian online, April 2011. *http://www.guardian.co.uk/science/2011/apr/07/antibiotic-resistance-bacteria?INTCMP=SRCH*

57. Boseley S, Antibiotics' efficiency wanes due to global spread of drug-resistant bacteria. UK Guardian online, Aug 2010. *http://www.guardian.co.uk/science/2010/aug/11/antibiotics-efficiency-drug-resistant-bacteria?INTCMP=SRCH*

The Antibiotic Syndrome

58. Last W, Candida and the Antibiotic Syndrome. Health-Science-Spirit online. *http://www.health-science-spirit.com/candida.html*

Anti-Candida Diet

59. Crook WG, *The Yeast Connection and the Woman*, Professional Books: Jackson, TN, 1995.

60. Horowitz BJ, et al, Sugar chromatography studies in recurrent candida vulvovaginitis. *J Reprod Med*; 29(7): pp 441-3, July 1984. *http://www.ncbi.nlm.nih.gov/pubmed/6481700*

61. Cadieux P, et al, Lactobacillus strains and vaginal ecology. *JAMA*; 287(15): 1940-1941. *http://jama.jamanetwork.com/article.aspx?volume=287&issue=15&page=1940*

62. Wolfe I, Dr Crook's Candida Diet. Livestrong online, Sept 2011. *http://www.livestrong.com/article/537841-dr-crooks-candida-diet/*

63. Fitzsimmons, et al, Inhibition of Candida albicans by Lactobacillus acidophilus: Evidence for the involvement of a peroxidase system. *Microbios*; 80 (323): pp 125-33, 1994. *http://www.ncbi.nlm.nih.gov/pubmed/7898374*

64. William Crook's Candida Questionnaire. Flora-Balance.com online, excerpt from *The Yeast Connection Handbook*; Professional Books: Jackson, Tennessee, 2002. *http://www.flora-balance.com/candida_questionnaire_long.php*

Lugol's Iodine

65. J Crow's Material Safety Data Sheet for Lugol's Iodine Toxicity. J Crow's online, Oct 2012. *http://www.jcrows.com/msds2.pdf*

66. Brownstein D, *Iodine: Why You Need It, Why You Can't Live Without It*, Medical Alternative Press: West Bloomfield, MI, Fourth Edition, 2009.

67. Eby G, Iodine: The Candida Killer! Curezone online, Candida Forum, 2007. *http://curezone.com/forums/am.asp?i=859530*

68. Kariuki E, et al. Povidone iodine therapy for recurrent oral Candidiasis to prevent emerging Antifungal resistant Candida Strains. *Int Conf AIDS*; pp 9-14; 13: abstract no. MoPeB2281, July 2000. *http://iodine4health.com/disease/candida/kariuki_candida.htm*

69. Bhatt BM, et al, Suppression of Mixed Candida Biofilms with an Iodine Oral Rinse. Biomedical Development Corporation online, San Antonio, TX, USA; The University of Texas Health Science Center at San Antonio, March 2007. *http://iadr.confex.com/iadr/2007orleans/techprogram/abstract_90538.htm*

70. Waltimo TM, et al, In vitro susceptibility of Candida albicans to four disinfectants and their combinations. *Intl Endodontic Journal*; 32 (6); pp 421–429, Nov 1999. *http://onlinelibrary.wiley.com/doi/10.1046/j.1365-2591.1999.00237.x/abstract?userIsAuthenticated=false&deniedAccessCustomisedMessage=*

71. Shormon M, Candidiasis Yeast Overgrowth and Thyroid Disease. About.com online, 2003. *http://thyroid.about.com/cs/relatedconditions/a/candida.htm*

72. Winkler R, Iodine effects in body tissues - a survey and biophysical approach to interpretation. *Wien Klin Wochenschr*, 88 (13): pp 405-12, June 1976. *http://www.ncbi.nlm.nih.gov/pubmed/983067?dopt=AbstractPlus*

73. Last W, WARNING: IODINE IN LUGOL'S SOLUTION. Health-Science-Spirit online. *http://www.health-science-spirit.com/lugol.htm*

Optimox Research: The Iodine Utilization Project

74. Abraham GE, The Wolff-Chaikoff Effect: Crying Wolf? *The Original Internist*, 12 (3): 112-118, 2005. *http://www.optimox.com/pics/Iodine/pdfs/IOD04.pdf*

75. Abraham GE et al, Orthoiodosupplementation: Iodine Sufficiency Of The Whole Human Body. *The Original Internist*, 9: pp 5-20, 2002. *http://www.optimox.com/pics/Iodine/IOD-02/IOD_02.htm*

76. Abraham GE, et al, Optimum Levels of Iodine for Greatest Mental and Physical Health. *The Original Internist*, 2002. *http://www.optimox.com/pics/Iodine/pdfs/IOD01.pdf*

77. Abraham, GE, The History of Iodine in Medicine Part I: From Discovery to Essentiality. *The Original Internist*, 13: pp 29-36, Spring 2006. *http://www.hakalalabs.com/Research/Abraham_OI_Spring06.pdf*

78. Abraham GE, The History of Iodine in Medicine Part II: The Search for and the Discovery of Thyroid Hormones. *The Original Internist*, 13: pp 67-70, June 2006. *http://www.hakalalabs.com/Research/Abraham_OI_Jun06_1.pdf*

79. Abraham GE, The History of Iodine in Medicine Part III: Thyroid Fixation and Medical Iodophobia. *The Original Internist*, 13: pp 71-78, June 2006. *http://www.hakalalabs.com/Research/Abraham_OI_Jun06_2.pdf*

80. Abraham GE, et al, Effect of daily ingestion of a tablet containing 5 mg iodine and 7.5 mg iodide as the potassium salt, for a period of 3 months, on the results of thyroid function tests and thyroid volume by ultrasonometry in ten euthyroid Caucasian women. *The Original Internist*, 9: pp 6-20 March 2008. *http://www.hakalalabs.com/Research/Abraham_OI_Mar08.pdf*

81. Abraham GE, Facts about Iodine and Autoimmune Thyroiditis. *The Original Internist*, 15 (2), pp 75-76, June 2008. *http://www.hakalalabs.com/Research/Abraham_OI_Jun08.pdf*

The Iodine Protocol

82. The Iodine Protocol with Companion Nutrients. Breast Cancer Choices online. *http://www.breastcancerchoices.org/iprotocol.html*

83. Abraham GE, et al, The Safe and Effective Implementation of Ortho-iodo-supplementation. In Medical Practice, Fibromyalgia Recovery online. PowerPoint presentation. *http://fibromyalgiarecovery.com/uploads/IODINE_-_Solution_to_health_problems.pdf*

Neutrophil Research

84. Iodine and the Body. Iodine Research online. Various research articles. *http://www.iodineresearch.com/immunepg1.html*

Turpentine/Kerosene vs Candida

85. Daniels J, The Candida Cleaner. Yahoo Groups online. *http://xa.yimg.com/kq/groups/11136827/2098715122/name/Turpentine-The_Candida_Cleaner+-Dr.+Daniels.pdf*

86. Last W, Kerosene – A Universal Healer. Health-Science-Spirit online. *http://www.health-science-spirit.com/kero.htm*

87. Kerosene and Cancer, Rethinking Cancer online. F.A.C.T. article. *http://www.rethinkingcancer.org/resources/magazine-articles/7_9-10/kerosene.php*

88. Mercier B, et al, The Essential Oil of Turpentine and its Major Volatile Faction alpha-and beta-pinenes: A Review. *Intl Jour of Occ Med and Envir Health*; 22(4): pp 331–342; 89. 2009. *http://www.imp.lodz.pl/upload/oficyna/artykuly/pdf/full/--04_09_Mercier.pdf*

89. Rivas da Silva AC, et al, Biological activities of α-pinene and β-pinene enantiomers. *Molecules*; 25; 17(6): pp 6305-16; May 2012. *http://www.ncbi.nlm.nih.gov/pubmed/22634841*

Magnesium

90. Last W, Magnesium Chloride for Health & Rejuvenation. Nexus Magazine online, Nov 2008. *http://www.health-science-spirit.com/magnesiumchloride.html*

Borax Boron

91. Last W, The Borax Conspiracy. Health-Science-Spirit online. *http://www.health-science-spirit.com/borax.htm*

92. Last W, The Ultimate Cleanse. Health-Science-Spirit online. *http://www.health-science-spirit.com/ultimatecleanse.html*

93. Newham RE, et al, The Art of Getting Well: Boron and Arthritis. The Arthritis Trust of America online, 1994. *http://www.arthritistrust.org/Articles/Boron%20and%20Arthritis.pdf*

Vitamin C

94. Klenner FR, Massive doses of vitamin C and the virus diseases. *South Med Surg.*; 113 (4): pp 101-7; 1951. *http://pmid.us/14855098.*

95. Cathcart RF, Vitamin C, titrating to bowel tolerance, anascorbemia, and acute induced scurvy. *Med Hypotheses*; 7(11): pp 1359-76; 1981. *http://pmid.us/7321921*

96. Cathcart RF, A unique function for ascorbate. *Med Hypotheses*; 35 (1): pp 32-7; May 1991. *http://pmid.us/1921774*

97. Thomas WR, et al, Vitamin C and immunity: an assessment of the evidence. *Clin Exp Immunol*; 32 (2): pp 370-9; May 1978. *http://pmid.us/352590.*

98. Nandi BK, et al, Effect of ascorbic acid on detoxification of histamine under stress conditions. *Biochem Pharmacol*; 1;23 (3): pp 643-7; Feb 1974. *http://pmid.us/4132605.*

99. Furuya A, et al, Antiviral effects of ascorbic and dehydroascorbic acids in vitro. *Int J Mol Med*; 22 (4): pp 541-5; Oct 2008. *http://pmid.us/18813862.*

100. Riordan HD et al, A pilot clinical study of continuous intravenous ascorbate in terminal cancer patients. *PR Health Sci J*; 24 (4): pp 269-76; Dec. 2005. *http://pmid.us/16570523*

101. Hoffer LJ, et al. Ascorbic acid in advanced malignancy. *Ann. Oncol*; 19 (11): 1969-74. *http://pmid.us/18544557.*

102. Andreasen CB, et al, The effects of ascorbic acid on in vitro heterophil function. *Avian Dis*; 43 (4): pp 656-63. Oct-Dec 1999. *http://pmid.us/10611981.*

Alpha Lipoic Acid

103. Berkson B, *The Alpha Lipoic Acid Breakthrough*; Three Rivers Press: New York, 1995.

104. Rogers SA, Lipoic Acid as a Potential First Agent for Protection from Mycotoxins and Treatment of Mycotoxicosis. *Arch. Of Env. Health*; 58 (8); pp 528-532; 2003. *http://www.tandfonline.com/doi/abs/10.3200/AEOH.58.8.528-532*

Selenium

105. Boyne R, Arthur JR, The response of Selenium deficient mice to Candida Albicans infection. *Journ. Of Nutrition*; 116 (5): pp 816-822; 1986. *http://europepmc.org/abstract/MED/3701459*

106. Manavathu M, et al, Changes in glutathione metabolize enzymes during yeast-to-mycelium conversion of Candida albicans. *Can J Microbiol*; 42 (1): pp 76-9; Jan 1996. *http://www.ncbi.nlm.nih.gov/pubmed/8595600*

107. Black A, The mineral selenium proves itself as powerful anti-cancer medicine. Natural News online, Jan 2009. *http://www.naturalnews.com/016446_selenium_nutrition.html*

108. Mazokopakis EE, et al, Effects of 12 months treatment with L-selenomethionine on serum anti-TPO Levels in Patients with Hashimoto's thyroiditis. *Thyroid*; 17 (7): pp 609-12; July 2007. *http://www.ncbi.nlm.nih.gov/pubmed/17696828*

109. Gartner R, et al, Selenium Supplementation in Patients with Autoimmune Thyroiditis Decreases Thyroid Peroxidase Antibodies Concentrations. *The Jour of Clin Endo & Metab*; 87(4): pp 1687-1691; Jan 2002. *http://integrativehealthconnection.com/wp-content/uploads/2011/11/Selenium-Supplementation-in-Patients-with-Autoimmune-Thyroiditis-Decreases-Thyroid-Peroxidase-Antibodies-Concentrations.pdf*

110. Dach J, Selenium for Hashimoto's Thyroiditis. Natural Thyroid Blog online, Sep 2011. *http://jdach1.typepad.com/natural_thyroid/2011/02/selenium-for-hashimotos-thyroiditis-by-jeffrey-dach-md.html*

B Vitamins

111. Saul A, et al, *Niacin: The Real Story*; Basic Health Publications Inc.: Laguna Beach, CA, 2012.

112. Eaton KK, et al, Abnormal gut fermentation laboratory studies reveal deficiency of B-vitamins, zinc and magnesium, *J Nutr Biochem*; 4 (11); pp 635–638; 1993. *http://www.sciencedirect.com/science/article/pii/095528639390035U*

113. Vitamin B3 May Offer New Tool in Fight Against Staph Infections, 'Superbugs'. Science Daily online, Aug 2012. *http://www.sciencedaily.com/releases/2012/08/120827122258.htm*

114. Kyme P, et al, C/EBPε mediates nicotinamide-enhanced clearance of Staphylococcus aureus in mice. *J Clin Invest*; 122 (9): pp 3316–3329; 2012. *http://www.jci.org/articles/view/62070*

115. Fassa P, Niacin is a Booster Rocket for Detoxification, Natural News online, July 2011. *http://www.naturalnews.com/033168_niacin_detoxification.html*

Alkalizing the Body

116. Napatalung P, Thompson B, *pH Balanced for Life!: The Easiest Way to Alkalize*; Earth Clinic Publications, Body Axis LLC: Atlanta, 2012.

Fulvic/Humic Acid

117. Sherry L, et al, Carbohydrate Derived Fulvic Acid: An in vitro Investigation of a Novel Membrane Active Antiseptic Agent Against Candida albicans Biofilms. *Front Microbiol*, 3: 116; 2012. http://www.ncbi.nlm.nih.gov/pubmed/22479260

118. Fulvic acid and its use in the treatment of candida infections. Free Patents Online. *European Patent Specification, Patent ref: EP1700599 B1*; Oct 8, 1999. http://www.freepatentsonline.com/EP1700599.pdf

119. Morales OY, et al, Fulvic Acid and Viral Infections. *Open Conf Proc Journal*, 3; pp 24-29; 2012. http://benthamscience.com/open/toprocj/articles/V003/24TOPROCJ.pdf

120. Dekker J, Fulvic acid and its use in the treatment of viral infections. FPO online, *European Patent, Patent ref: EP1698333*, Oct 8, 2008. https://www.siselinternational.com/cms-science/US/en/Fulvic_Acid_References.pdf

Zinc

121. Sterniolo GC, et al, Zinc supplementation tightens "leaky gut" in Crohn's disease. *Inflammatory Bowel Disease*; 7 (2); pp 94–98; May 2001. http://onlinelibrary.wiley.com/doi/10.1097/00054725-200105000-00003/full

Green Tea

122. Hirasawa M, et al, Multiple effects of green tea catechin on the antifungal activity of antimycotics against Candida albicans, *J Antimicrob Chemother*, 53 (2): pp 2259; Feb 2004. http://www.ncbi.nlm.nih.gov/pubmed/14688042

123. Evensen NA, et al, The effects of tea polyphenols on Candida albicans: inhibition of biofilm formation and proteasome inactivation. *Can J Microbiol*, 55 (9): pp 1033-9; Sep 2009. http://www.ncbi.nlm.nih.gov/pubmed/19898545

Pau D'Arco

124. Höfling JF, et al, Antimicrobial potential of some plant extracts against Candida species. *J Antimicib Chemother*, 53(2): pp 225-9; Feb 2004. http://www.ncbi.nlm.nih.gov/pubmed/21180915

125. Melo e Silva, F, et al. Evaluation of the antifungal potential of Brazilian Cerrado medicinal plants. *Mycoses*; 52 (6): pp 511-7; 1439-0507; Nov 2009. *http://www.ncbi.nlm.nih.gov/pubmed/19207849*

126. Pereira, EM, et al. Tabebuia avellanedae naphthoquinones: activity against methicillin-resistant staphylococcal strains, cytotoxic activity and in vivo dermal irritability analysis. *Ann. Clin. Microbiol. Antimicrob*; 5 (5); Mar 2006. *http://www.ann-clinmicrob.com/content/5/1/5;* Portillo A., et al. Antifungal activity of Paraguayan plants used in traditional medicine. *J. Ethnopharmacol*; 76 (1): 93–8; Jun 2001. *http://www.ncbi.nlm.nih.gov/pubmed/12636992*

127. Park, BS, et al. Antibacterial activity of Tabebuia impetiginosa Martius ex DC Taheebo against Helicobacter pylori. *J. Ethnopharmacol*; 105 1-2: pp 255-62; April 2006. *http://www.ncbi.nlm.nih.gov/pubmed/16359837*

128. Park, BS, et al, Selective growth-inhibiting effects of compounds identified in Tabebuia impetiginosa inner bark on human intestinal bacteria. *J. Agric. Food Chem*; 53 (4): pp 1152-7; Feb 2005. *http://www.ncbi.nlm.nih.gov/pubmed/15713033*

129. Machado TB, et al. In vitro activity of Brazilian medicinal plants, naturally occurring naphthoquinones and their analogues, against methicillin-resistant Staphylococcus aureus. *Int. J. Antimicrob. Agents*; 21 (3): 279-84; 2003. *http://www.sciencedirect.com/science/article/pii/S0924857902003497*

130. Nagata K., et al. Antimicrobial activity of novel furanonaphthoquinone analogs. *Antimicrobial Agents Chemother*; 42 (3): 700–2; 1998. *http://aac.asm.org/content/42/3/700.full.pdf*

131. Binutu OA, et al. Antimicrobial potentials of some plant species of the Bignoniaceae family. *Afr. J. Med. Sci.*; 23 3: 269–73; 1994. *http://www.ncbi.nlm.nih.gov/pubmed/7604753*

132. Giuraud P., et al. Comparison of antibacterial and antifungal activities of lapachol and b-lapachone. *Planta Med*; 60 (4): 373–74; Aug 1994. *http://www.ncbi.nlm.nih.gov/pubmed/7938274*

Nystatin Antifungal

133. Nystatin: Prescribing Information. WHO online, WHO Model Prescribing Information (HIV), 2013. *http://apps.who.int/medicinedocs/en/d/Js2215e/9.19.html*

134. Nystatin: Sigma-Aldritch Product Information. Sigma-Aldrich online. 2013. *http://www.sigmaaldrich.com/etc./medialib/docs/Sigma/Product_Information_Sheet/2/n6261pis.Par.0001.File.tmp/n6261pis.pdf*

Biofilm Removal with Protease Enzymes (Fibrinolytic Enzymes)

135. Cohen P, Interview with Dr Cohen concerning biofilms and enzyme therapies. Lafora Free Forum online, Jan 2011. *http://pptu.lefora.com/2011/01/17/interview-with-dr-cohen-concerning-biofilms-and-en/*

136. Hisanori Akiyama, et al, Biofilm formation of Staphylococcus aureus strains isolated from impetigo and furuncle: role of fibrinogen and fibrin. *Jour of Dermatol. Sc.*; 16 (1); pp 2-10; Nov 1997. *http://www.sciencedirect.com/science/article/pii/S0923181197006117*

137. Kelly G, Bromelain: A Literature Review and Discussion of its Therapeutic Applications. *ALT MED Rev*; 1 (4): 243-257; 1996. *http://www.thorne.com/altmedrev/.fulltext/1/4/243.pdf*

138. Maurer HR, Bromelain: biochemistry, pharmacology and medical use. *Cell. Mol. Life Sci. 58*; pp 1234–1245; Mar 2001. *http://www.volopharm.de/daten/Bromelain%20biochemistry,%20pharmacology%20and%20medical%20use.pdf*

Molybdenum vs Candida

139. Schmitt DC Jr, et al, The Art of Getting Well: Molybdenum for Candida and Other Problems. Arthritis Trust online, 1991. *http://www.arthritistrust.org/Articles/Molybdenum%20for%20Candida%20albicans%20Patients.pdf*

ABOUT THE AUTHOR

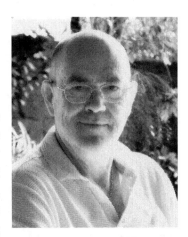

Bill Thompson

Bill Thompson entered the Earth Clinic community years ago as one of the walking unwell but has emerged not only wholly well but furthermore as an expert in alternative therapies. In particular, Mr. Thompson has established an eager following for his advice on alkalizing techniques and the treatment of systemic candida—two areas of complementary healthcare he has studied extensively and in successful application to his own health.

After a productive career as a software analyst and entrepreneur, Bill Thompson was able to enter into an early retirement in the Philippines, where he could launch into this second lifetime in alternative health. The analytical skills required by his first career and life-long interest in natural herbal therapies have made him the perfect counselor to weigh the evidence both for and against powerful natural remedies, and to present them cogently to a world of people eager for inexpensive, natural medicines.

Mr. Thompson, now in his sixties, enjoys the company of his family and the successes of his two grown sons.

Discover other Earth Clinic titles at EarthClinic.com
Apple Cider Vinegar: A Modern Folk Remedy
Nature's Best Remedies
pH Balanced for Health: The Easiest Way to Alkalize

Connect with Us Online!
https://twitter.com/ - !/Earth_Clinic
http://www.facebook.com/pages/Earth-Clinic/60803892726

Printed in Great Britain
by Amazon.co.uk, Ltd.,
Marston Gate.